FAST FACTS FOR THE MEDICAL OFFICE NURSE

What You Really Need to Know in a Nutshell

D0873529

Sheila Richmeier, MS, RN, FACMPE, is a practice enhancement facilitator for TransforMED, a subsidiary of the American Academy of Family Physicians, where she facilitates the adoption of the Patient Centered Medical Home for primary care practices. She has a rich background in multiple settings as a practice administrator and clinician. Her experience includes hospital and community settings (home health, urgent care, consulting, education, and medical offices). Sheila graduated with her masters in nursing administration from the University of Kansas School of Nursing. She is a fellow in the American College of Medical Practice Executives and is board certified by ANCC in Community Health Nursing. She has published two books, *Leading Your Clinical Team: A Comprehensive Guide to Optimizing Productivity and Quality* (2009) and *The New Healthcare Supervisor's Guide: The Secret to Success* (2010). She was also a co-author on a national study on the nursing shortage, published by AJN. As a current member of MGMA, KMGMA, and GKCMMA, she has served in various leadership roles in nursing and practice management organizations. Sheila has entertained various national speaking engagements as an expert in clinical efficiency and staffing, patient-centered medical home management, and practice management. She can be contacted at Sheila-Richmeier@att.net.

FAST FACTS FOR THE MEDICAL OFFICE NURSE

What You Really Need to Know in a Nutshell

Sheila Richmeier, MS, RN, FACMPE

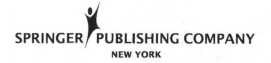

SPRINGER PUBLISHING COMPANY
NEW YORK

BP45

Springer Publishing Company, LLC
11 West 42nd Street
New York, NY 10036
www.springerpub.com

Acquisitions Editor: Allan Graubard
Project Editor: Gayle Lee
Cover Design: David Levy
Composition: Ashita Shah at Newgen Imaging Systems Ltd.

ISBN: 978–0–8261–0679–7
E-book ISBN: 978–0–8261–0680–3

10 11 12/ 5 4 3 2 1

The author and the publisher of this Work have made every effort to use sources believed to be reliable to provide information that is accurate and compatible with the standards generally accepted at the time of publication. Because medical science is continually advancing, our knowledge base continues to expand. Therefore, as new information becomes available, changes in procedures become necessary. We recommend that the reader always consult current research and specific institutional policies before performing any clinical procedure. The author and publisher shall not be liable for any special, consequential, or exemplary damages resulting, in whole or in part, from the readers' use of, or reliance on, the information contained in this book. The publisher has no responsibility for the persistence or accuracy of URLs for external or third-party Internet Web sites referred to in this publication and does not guarantee that any content on such Web sites is, or will remain, accurate or appropriate.

Library of Congress Cataloging-in-Publication Data

Richmeier, Sheila.
   Fast facts for the medical office nurse : what you really need to know in a nutshell / Sheila Richmeier.
      p. ; cm.
   Includes bibliographical references and index.
   ISBN 978–0–8261–0679–7 (alk. paper)
   1. Medical office nursing. I. Title.
   [DNLM: 1. Office Nursing. WY 109 R532f 2010]
   RT120.O9R53   2010
   610.73—dc22
                                                                      2010012396

Printed in the United States of America by Hamilton Printing.

2/23/11

Contents

Foreword

Every job is a self-portrait of the one who did it—
autograph your work with excellence!

Author Unknown

In nursing school, I had many conversations with my
peers about what kind of nursing we wanted to explore
when we graduated. The most popular picks were mother/
baby, surgery, intensive care...nursing homes were at the
bottom of the list, and office nursing didn't even show up
on the radar! After graduation, my experience as a nurse
grew, and I found myself working in a multispecialty/
multiphysician clinic as a float nurse.

With more than 60 offices in this clinic, I walked in
fear of the physicians' wrath and kept a notebook detail-
ing information about how each physician wanted things
done—even down to how they wanted the chart placed
in the holder outside of the room! I had lost my professional compass and had slipped into a mindless excuse
for a nurse. Instead of seeing an exciting opportunity to
make a difference and affect the lives of the patients, I
wallowed in drudgery. Instead of assisting the physicians
in making their practice all that it could be, I allowed

myself to become a plodder and shamefully fulfill the demeaning concept of, "Oh, she's *just* an office nurse."

It didn't help that some physicians had a "nurse-is-a-nurse-is-a-nurse" mentality. Some "nurses" were not licensed nurses—just "wanna-bes" the physician had trained. The line between the licensed and nonlicensed nursing staff had blurred.

Enter Sheila. While using her as a sounding board, our conversation traveled into the realm of constructive brainstorming. We engaged in some friendly but very heated conversations about what office nursing should and could be. Out of this "storm" grew a plan; from a plan, grew action and results.

With input from other nurses, physicians, and administrative staff, we were able to create a professional nursing presence, empower the licensed nursing staff, and provide training to nonlicensed staff. The ultimate benefactors were the patients and clients.

Professional nursing, *regardless of the milieu*, is the *most important nursing you will ever do.* As office nurses, you will have your own set of issues, hurdles, and challenges. Embrace them! You *are* a critical thinker, not a trained automaton. You are not a gatekeeper! You are the first professional contact in the health care setting. Proudly step up to the plate!

Karla Arbuckle, RN, BSN
Special Education School Nurse,
Reno County Education Cooperative
Interlocal District 610

Preface

Over the years, medical office nursing has been seen as the kind of nursing that would be sought after many years of experience as a nurse. It was a slower pace and it didn't require the skills and competencies of hospital nursing. In fact, in many cases it was believed that nurses in the medical office could no longer "cut it" in the hospital. There was never any care provided in a medical office; it was just a place where patients saw their physicians. Nurses played a subservient role, and the role of handmaiden was seen as below the standards of "real" nurses.

This book takes those misconceptions and blows them to bits. Medical office nursing is not only high-tech at times, but it is very much high-touch. Nurses are needed in medical offices to provide high-quality care to keep patients out of the hospital, maximize patient outcomes, and reduce costs.

The transition to a medical office nurse is not easy for some since the skills and duties required may have never been encountered in other settings. This book may give you a head start on medical office skills, and can be used as a reference in the future when you encounter a new situation in the medical office.

Medical office nursing was a pivotal position for me in my career. After numerous years in the hospital and home health care industries, I took a position as an urgent care supervisor in a multispecialty clinic. I became fascinated with the knowledge and skill of the medical office nurses and learned as much from them as I could. Medical office nursing also laid the foundation for my future role as a medical practice manager and consultant. Today I help practices throughout the country optimize their offices, and an efficient medical office nursing staff is a big part of it. I would like to take you on a journey through understanding and starting a career in medical office nursing.

Sheila Richmeier, MS, RN, FACMPE

Acknowledgments

I would like to recognize all of my past coworkers, supervisors, and practices that I have worked with that have helped me gain further knowledge of medical office nursing. I have been told that when you see one practice, you see one practice. That is so true with medical office nursing, and the more nursing staffs I encounter, the more I learn about what a great profession medical office nursing is. There is no right or wrong way to do this, but thanks to the dedication of nurses in many offices, there is a better way to provide excellent nursing care. I commend all of them for the work that they do and you for the work you will do as a new medical office nurse. A special thanks to the staff at TransforMED to allow me to learn so much from them and continue the great work of transformation in medical practices.

Introduction

INTRODUCTION

This chapter will give an introduction to what medical office nursing is and can be. We start with a questionnaire, which demonstrates some key points you will learn as you read the book.

In this chapter, you will learn:

1. The different components of medical office nursing.
2. An understanding of the book's content.

Medical office nursing is quite different from other types of nursing and requires you to use your current skills and learn new ones. Throughout this book those skills are further clarified as medical office nursing is explained and components of the career are explored. Some chapters might make your head spin as we talk about subjects you, as a nurse, may not have been exposed to previously, such as coding and reimbursement. Hang in there—many nurses have learned it and then said, "It's not that bad." The following questionnaire will get you started.

QUESTIONNAIRE

Answer "T" for true and "F" for false for the following questions to see what you currently know about medical office nursing. Then review the brief answers that follow the questionnaire.

1. The physician's office is the only location for medical office nursing.
2. Evaluation and management is one type of care provided in the medical office.
3. CPT stands for computerized physician technology.
4. Medical office nurses will never need to understand billing and coding.
5. Ambulatory care is care provided in an upright position.
6. Nurses will use the practice management system often.
7. Patients can communicate with the practice using the patient portal.
8. Nurse practitioners can assist the physician with health assessments as well as nursing home and hospital rounds.
9. Medication management is the sole responsibility of the physician.
10. Measuring outcomes can improve patient care.
11. Patient satisfaction is an outcome that is measured in a medical office.

12. With training, the medical assistant can become a valued member of the team.
13. One way to reduce phone volume is to ask the patients not to call.
14. Pharmaceutical representatives are always welcomed into the practice.
15. The future of medical office nursing is vast, creating a truly rewarding career.

ANSWERS TO THE QUESTIONS

1. The physician's office is the only location for medical office nursing.
False. There are many locations for medical office nursing. This book concentrates on the physician's medical office, but all the concepts could be applied to other settings. Medical office nursing is a form of ambulatory nursing, and Chapter 2 will discuss locations and common themes for every medical office.

FAST FACTS in a NUTSHELL

A medical office nurse can work in many different locations.

2. Evaluation and management is one type of care provided in the medical office.
True. Evaluation and management is one type of care provided by physicians, nurse practitioners, and even

registered nurses in a medical office setting. Understanding the types of services will give you a good idea about how your role fits into a medical office. In Chapter 2 we will explore all the services provided in a medical office.

===*FAST FACTS in a NUTSHELL*

Evaluation and management is a type of service provided in a medical office.

3. CPT stands for computerized physician technology.
False. CPT stands for Current Procedure Technology, and is used for identifying and coding different types of services. You will use CPT often as a medical office nurse. The explanation of how services are paid for included in Chapter 3 may be complicated, but with a little use will become second nature.

===*FAST FACTS in a NUTSHELL*

Coding is one of the responsibilities of a medical office nurse.

4. Medical office nurses will never need to understand billing and coding.
False. In order for you to fully carry out your duties as a medical office nurse, you will need to learn some basic coding and billing rules. Unlike hospital nursing, medical office nursing requires the nurse to be a part of the billing mechanism for

the practice. However, with that being said, there are many resources that you can tap into to enable you to function. Chapter 3 will give you an overview of billing and coding.

═══════════════════════════*FAST FACTS in a NUTSHELL*

Medical office nursing requires a basic understanding of coding and billing.

5. Ambulatory care is care provided in an upright position.

False. Although in some cases care could be provided in an upright position, ambulatory care is provided on an outpatient basis instead of an inpatient basis. Ambulatory care is the all-encompassing care provided outside of the hospital setting. Medical office nursing is just one of the types of ambulatory care that is provided. In Chapter 4, the different facets of patient care and how ambulatory care fits into the overall health care arena will be explored.

═══════════════════════════*FAST FACTS in a NUTSHELL*

Outpatient care is a characteristic of ambulatory care.

6. Nurses will use the practice management system often.

True. As a medical office nurse, you will need to be aware of the physician's schedule at all times, and scheduling is part of the practice management system. You will also access some billing functions when you talk to insurance companies; thus, billing is a big part of the practice management system. Chapter 5 will discuss technology and how the medical office nurse uses such technology.

================ *FAST FACTS in a NUTSHELL*

- Technology and software programs will be different for the medical office nurse.
- They will include billing and scheduling programs.

7. Patients can communicate with the practice using the patient portal.

True. New technology using electronic communication is rapidly gaining traction in medical offices. Access to care is about providing a means for patients to communicate about their health care condition. In Chapter 5, new technology will be discussed.

================ *FAST FACTS in a NUTSHELL*

Patients are using technology more and more to communicate with the medical office.

8. Nurse practitioners can assist the physician with health assessments as well as nursing home and hospital rounds.

True. These are a few of the many functions that a nurse practitioner can provide in a medical office. Nurse practitioners are becoming a bigger part of the provider structure due to physician shortages in primary care and other specialties. Nurse practitioners play a big role in supplementing and providing a wider range of services for a physician. The nurse practitioner and other roles in the medical office will be further explored in Chapter 6.

====================================*FAST FACTS in a NUTSHELL*

Nurse practitioners play a major role in medical offices.

9. Medication management is the sole responsibility of the physician.
False. Medication management is both a physician duty and a nursing duty. As a medical office nurse, you will be responsible to ensure that patients are taking the right medications, and you will also be asked to administer medications as part of your role. Physicians, of course, have the ultimate responsibility, but nurses play a large part in this. The many components of nursing roles in a medical office will be explored in Chapter 6.

====================================*FAST FACTS in a NUTSHELL*

Medication management is a major part of the nurse's role in medical office nursing.

10. Measuring outcomes can improve patient care.
True. Outcomes are becoming a bigger priority in all specialties. If we could not prove that our care maintained or improved the patient's health, why would we continue to

provide it? The measurement of various types of outcomes in a medical office is discussed in depth in Chapter 7.

════════════════════════════*FAST FACTS in a NUTSHELL*

- Providing quality care is proven with the measurement of clinical outcomes.
- Medical offices are measuring more and more outcomes.

11. Patient satisfaction is an outcome that is measured in a medical office.
True. Patient satisfaction used to be the only outcome that was measured in a medical office. Insurers, employers, employees, and providers are demanding more proof that care was provided and that the care had an impact on the patient's health. However, patient satisfaction is still a key outcome that allows the practice to understand from the patient's perspective how the care was provided. Satisfaction outcomes will be explained in Chapter 7.

════════════════════════════*FAST FACTS in a NUTSHELL*

- One quality outcome is patient satisfaction.
- Patient satisfaction outcomes provide a patient's perspective.

12. With training, the medical assistant can become a valued member of the team.
True. Medical assistants can become a valued member of the team and improve their skills through additional training

in specific procedures and processes. Your role as a nurse in the office will be to supervise and delegate appropriately to the nonlicensed staff. In Chapter 8, the role of the nurse is further defined and nonlicensed staff roles are clarified.

═══════════════════════*FAST FACTS in a NUTSHELL*

Medical assistants are used in the medical office to supplement the care of the physician and nurse.

13. One way to reduce phone volume is to ask patients not to call.
True, but you may be looking for a new job. Phone call volume can be high in many medical office settings, and any action that can reduce this volume is appreciated. For example, having the person who rooms the patient ask about refills will reduce the phone calls from the patients who have just seen the physician. In Chapter 8, other tips will be given to maximize the nurse's role in the medical office.

═══════════════════════*FAST FACTS in a NUTSHELL*

- Phone call volume is high in most medical offices.
- Tips to maximize the nurse's role will help reduce phone call volume.

14. Pharmaceutical representatives are always welcomed into the practice.
True and false. This is becoming less and less true. Pharmaceutical representatives want to talk with

physicians in order to educate them about their medications (and hopefully sell them), and physicians often discover new medications from pharmaceutical representatives. It is not uncommon for a medical practice to have thirty to forty representatives who call on them on a regular basis. Although pharmaceutical reps often provide lunch and samples, they are being allowed less and less access to the physician, and their visits are limited. How to manage pharmaceutical representatives and other tips will be given in Chapter 8.

======*FAST FACTS in a NUTSHELL*

- Pharmaceutical representatives visit physician offices to sell their products to physicians.
- Physicians are allowing them access less often.

15. The future of medical office nursing is vast, creating a truly rewarding career.
True. Medical office nursing is an exciting career, and it can be very rewarding for those who choose it. The role of the nurse is expanding as physicians realize nurses are a vital member of the team. Chapter 9 explores different possibilities for medical office nursing.

======*FAST FACTS in a NUTSHELL*

- Medical office nursing is an exciting career.
- The role is expanding.

This has been just a taste of what you will learn as you move through this book. Each of the above subjects will be further explored and others will be explained. Now you are ready to begin learning about medical office nursing, with all of its differences, challenges, and joys. Enjoy this book and use it as a reference later as needed.

2

Medical Office Location and Care Provided

INTRODUCTION

Medical office services can be provided in multiple locations, and with each location, similarities are found. A medical office is a setting in which various services can be provided. This chapter will explore those services and how the nursing role is affected.

In this chapter, you will learn:

1. Three common themes for all medical offices.
2. What care is provided in the medical office setting.
3. The nurse's role in providing services.

LOCATION OF SERVICES

Medical services can be performed in many different settings. A medical office brings to mind a picture of Marcus Welby standing in his office taking care of patients. Numerous variations of that theme include:

- Private physician office
- Multispecialty clinic
- Private nurse practitioner office
- Urgent care clinic
- Surgical center
- Wound care clinic
- Health department
- Occupational health center
- Community care center
- Academic health center
- Hospital outpatient care

Although each of these examples is in a different location, all of them have this in common: a clinician is providing care to an individual in an outpatient setting. The clinician may vary from a physician to a nurse practitioner or from a nurse to an occupational therapist. The service may vary from wound care to evaluation and management of the patient's condition. However, one thing is true of all—a clinician is providing some type of care. Another thing is also true of all settings: The care is being provided to an individual, a patient, customer, or client. The last thing all of these settings have in common is that the care is provided outside the hospital or in an ambulatory care setting.

Services provided in the various settings may be different because of the clinician, the care that is provided, or the patient clientele. All settings provide medical services. The term "medical service" is an all-inclusive term that includes various types of care performed by a person trained in medicine or health care. Medical services could include

==*FAST FACTS in a NUTSHELL*

All medical office settings have three things in common:

1. A clinician
2. Care is provided
3. Outpatient setting

seeing patients, performing procedures, drawing blood for laboratory testing, providing diagnostic services, providing therapy services, or selling products. Services provided in a medical office will be further explored in the next sections of this chapter. These include evaluation and management, procedures, ancillary services, and care management.

EVALUATION AND MANAGEMENT

Evaluation and management (E&M) services refer to visits and consultations with nursing staff, physicians, and midlevel providers (nurse practitioners, physician assistants). A visit is a face-to-face meeting between the health care provider and the patient. E&M services are used extensively in all physicians' offices for new patient visits, preventive care, consults, and established patient visits. Physician hospital, nursing home, and home visits are also E&M. Specific examples of E&M visits include a three-month check-up for a diabetes patient, a sick visit for a child with a fever, a physical for a thirty-year-old, a hospital visit for a patient admitted for surgery, a yearly physician visit to a nursing home patient, and a first-time visit to a surgeon. Most visits in physicians' offices are for evaluation and management of the patient's condition.

===== *FAST FACTS in a NUTSHELL*

> Evaluation and management services include new and established patient visits, hospital and nursing home visits, preventive care visits, home visits, and nursing visits.

As you can see with the above examples, there are many reasons to see a physician in a medical office. Preventive visits include physicals, well-woman exams, and well-child exams. In contrast, a problem-focused exam could include chronic disease management every three to six months for a problem such as diabetes, hypertension, or cardiac disease, or an acute problem such as sore throat, back pain, ankle pain, or cough. A new patient visit may be for a preventive physical, an acute problem, or a chronic disease check. With the new patient visit, the patient has not been seen by this physician before. An established patient visit also may be preventive, acute, or for a chronic disease check; however, the established patient has been seen by the physician before.

Three components make up every E&M visit. During the course of the visit, the provider will evaluate the patient's history, conduct an examination, and make medical decisions related to the care of the patient.

The first step is obtaining a patient history. The patient's history includes the chief complaint, why the patient is here today, as well as the history of the present illness. The chief complaint is a statement describing the condition, symptom, problem, or diagnosis that brought the patient to the office. The history of present illness includes the following elements: location, quality, severity, duration, timing, context, modifying factors, and contributing signs and symptoms; and a review of all other pertinent systems, such as eyes, ears, cardiovascular, respiratory, gastrointestinal, genitourinary, musculoskeletal, integumentary, neurological, psychiatric, endocrine, hematologic, and allergic. A patient's past, family, and social history are also reviewed. The extent of the history is related to the provider's clinical judgment and the nature of the presenting problem.

Table 2.1 provides two examples of how the patient history is collected using the above elements. The first is a patient with ankle pain, and the second is a patient with a cough.

You can see that to document an E&M visit, many questions would be asked, some by the nurse and some by the physician. Knowing the actual history element used is not important. Knowing that history has to be taken, its importance, and the need for it to be as complete as possible is important, however.

The next part of the E&M visit is the physical exam. The physical exam varies, depending upon the chief complaint and the history elicited. In the first example, as you might expect, the physical exam would include

TABLE 2.1 Patient History		
History element	Patient 1	Patient 2
Chief complaint	Ankle pain	Cough
History of present illness		
Location	Left ankle	
Quality	Sharp pain	Productive cough
Severity	5 on a scale of 1 to 10	Cough produces yellow phlegm
Duration	Began 2 weeks ago	For 5 days
Timing	Has gotten worse in last 2 days	Worse at night
Context	More pain when standing	Short of breath with walking
Modifying factors	Ibuprofen lessens the pain to a 3 but does not relieve. Foot elevated brings some relief.	Using cough syrup without improvement
Contributing signs and symptoms	Swelling in ankle and foot	Fever and chest pain
Other pertinent systems		Nonsmoker
Past, family, and social history	Left ankle injury related to football in 2000	Bronchitis last year

examination of the left ankle and vital signs. In the second example, the physician would evaluate vital signs; listen to the heart and lungs; palpate neck lymph nodes; and look in the ears, nose, and throat.

The third step in the E&M visit is medical decision-making. Medical decision-making also varies, depending upon the chief complaint and the physical exam. In the first example above, the physician may order an x-ray to determine if there is a fracture, instruct the patient to elevate and apply ice packs, prescribe pain pills, and, if the ankle is not broken, refer the patient to the physical therapy department to evaluate and treat. In the second example, the physician may prescribe an antibiotic and an expectorant, do some lab work if indicated, and prescribe rest and relaxation. The medical decision-making is determined by the first two steps, history and exam.

The above two examples were for patients coming in with acute care needs. The same structure would be used for the chronic care visit. An example would be a patient seeing the doctor for a three-month diabetic follow-up visit. The history would revolve around the diabetes, the exam would supplement the history, and the medical decision-making would be the result of the findings from the history and the exam.

With a preventive care visit, the content and extent of a preventive exam is based on the patient's age, gender, and identified risk factors. The main focus of a preventive visit is to promote wellness and disease prevention. The visit may include additional testing or procedures such as Pap smears, vaccinations, screening lab testing, and counseling. The common denominators in a preventive visit are:

- Comprehensive history: This differs from the above history in that it is not problem-focused, but a comprehensive review of systems, past, family and social history, and pertinent risk factors
- Comprehensive physical: This is a multisystem exam based on age, gender, and identified risk factors
- Age-appropriate counseling and discussion of issues related to the specific age group: This may also include anticipatory guidance or review of safety issues, as well as the need for screening tests
- Appropriate immunizations or diagnostic tests or procedures
- Management of insignificant problems

Sometimes, the preventive visit can also include some problem-oriented services. For instance, the patient who is scheduled for a well-woman exam, which is a preventive service, also has a cold that is addressed by the physician. Depending upon the severity, this may turn into a problem-focused visit or a preventive/problem-focused visit. There are special coding requirements when this occurs.

Hospital, home, and nursing home visits follow the same guidelines. The clinician gathers a history, performs an exam, and makes medical decisions based on the exam. For instance, the hospital patient is admitted for chest pain. On the admission visit, the physician would take a complete history of this symptom, do an exam, and determine that the patient needs to be admitted to the hospital with many orders (i.e., the medical decision-making). On subsequent hospital visits, the physician will take a history of what has happened since he has last seen the patient, do an exam as needed, and make further medical decisions.

================*FAST FACTS in a NUTSHELL*

Evaluation and management codes are used with clinician office visits by evaluating the following:

* Patient's history
* Physical exam
* Medical decision-making

In a medical office, a nurse practitioner (NP) can provide E&M visits to any patient. Reimbursement may be less than the physician's visit due to the insurance company rules and regulations. Some insurance companies such as Medicare pay only 85 percent of the physician's usual fee for nurse practitioner's visits. Incident-to billing for Medicare allows the nurse practitioner services to be billed under the physician's number in certain situations and the reimbursement is at 100 percent of the physician fee schedule. The services have to be provided under the direct supervision of the physician (i.e., the physician must be present in the same office suite) and subsequent to the physician's establishment of the plan of care. Because of reimbursement issues, the office may restrict the nurse practitioner to certain visits to ensure optimal payment rates.

Nursing's role with E&M services is providing nursing visits, if applicable, which will be explained further in Chapter 3, and initiating the physician's visit by collecting elements of the history and exam. Nursing visits can be provided to evaluate and manage certain conditions. For provider visits, nursing will be collecting certain elements such as vital signs, chief complaint, and possibly some assessment items.

FAST FACTS in a NUTSHELL

A nurse's role with E&M visits is:

• Initiating collection of history elements
• Nursing visits

PROCEDURES

In this section, certain procedures will be discussed, including diagnostic, surgical, or other procedures performed by nurses. The different types of procedures depend upon the specialty and the physician's preference for the location of treatment. For instance, a surgeon may perform some procedures in the office and some in the hospital. Procedures that may be performed or scheduled by the medical office include:

• Minor surgical procedures: lesion removal, laceration repair, breast biopsy, toenail removal, cosmetic procedures

- Diagnostic procedures: sigmoidoscopy, bone marrow biopsy, punch needle biopsy, spinal tap, cardiac stress testing
- Nursing procedures: ear wash, urinary catheter exchange, injections, electrocardiogram (EKG), IV therapy, chemotherapy, central line flushing, colostomy bag change, spirometry
- Specialty surgical or diagnostic procedures: more complex procedures performed under anesthesia or a form of sedation

Procedures done outside the office will also have an impact on the nurse's role. For both types of procedures, tasks the nurse may be responsible for include:

- Managing the impact on the physician's office schedule
- Scheduling patients with other facilities
- Patient education before and after the procedure
- Insurance pre-authorization for the procedure
- Assisting with the procedure, including pre- and post-procedure work
- Follow-up phone calls

The nurse will be responsible for ensuring that the physician has adequate time to perform the procedure. She will also be involved in ensuring that the schedule has availability and is adequate for seeing patients prior to surgical procedures and for post-op care. Nursing staff schedule procedures in other facilities as well. Insurance pre-authorization for the procedure is another nursing role. This requires knowledge of the procedure and appropriate coding, and will be further explored in the next chapter.

Patient education entails an explanation of the procedure to supplement physician teaching, where and how it will be performed, and any preparation needed for the procedure. For instance, a colonoscopy will require a much different preparation than a breast biopsy. Educational resources could include preprinted literature or handouts the patient can review at a later time after they leave the office.

Another nursing role that relates to procedures may be to assist with the procedure, including pre- and post-op work. This can include setting up the sterile field, prepping the patient, positioning the patient appropriately, assisting the provider during the procedure, and then dressing the incision or assisting the patient to recover after the procedure.

Follow-up care may include: initiating post-op phone calls to patients who have had a procedure and answering questions regarding the procedure, side effects, or possible complications of the procedure; and assisting the billing staff with coding of the procedure.

FAST FACTS in a NUTSHELL

A nurse's role in caring for patients who are scheduled to have certain procedures include evaluating and managing the impact on the physician's

Continued

Continued

schedule, scheduling with other facilities, patient education, pre-authorizing the procedure, assisting the physician with the procedure both before and after, and follow-up care.

If you work with a physician who performs procedures outside of the office, it is important for you to understand, and perhaps watch, procedures so you can provide better patient education. You will be responsible for understanding that procedure and explaining it to the patient and/ or evaluating any post-operative complications. The more you know the actual steps in the process, the better you will be at explaining and working with the patient.

ANCILLARY SERVICES

Many offices provide some type of ancillary services. These can include:

- Lab testing
- Radiology
- Therapy (speech, occupational, or physical)
- Other diagnostic testing
- Retail outlet

Nursing's role in each of these is to understand when, why, and how they are ordered. Chances are the physician will come out of an exam room and give orders to the nursing staff to set up ancillary services. Most clinics have some capability to provide services on site. If not, nursing will direct patients to outside clinics.

Follow-up after any diagnostic test is important for many reasons: (a) it can be a liability issue if patients are not notified of their abnormal test results and (b) patients become more engaged in their care if they are fully informed of both normal and abnormal results. It is important to educate patients on why they should understand all test results. Test tracking to ensure all test results have been received can be done through a manual process or with the use of technology.

═══════════════════════════════*FAST FACTS in a NUTSHELL*

- Nursing's role with regard to ancillary services is to understand when, why, and how they are ordered.
- Follow-up care is important.

Listing all of the tests that were ordered for your patient and then knowing that the patient completed the test is the first step. A simple log can be created to start this tracking. The second step of tracking is knowing that the test results have been returned to the practice and that they have been reviewed. Once the review is complete, the third step is to notify the patient. Notification of lab results should include both normal and abnormal results. Some practices will tell the patient that "no news is good news" with regard to lab results notification. This can create a huge liability if the patient's results were abnormal and somehow the patient wasn't notified. This can be tracked on the log, and those test results that have not returned to the practice should be tracked down.

Electronic tracking can be used to signal that a test result has not been returned to the practice through the electronic medical record (EMR). A report can be run on a regular basis to ensure that all tests have been returned and that patients have been notified.

═══════════════════════════════*FAST FACTS in a NUTSHELL*

Test tracking is very important in a medical office:

- Track all tests by creating a log, manual or electronic.
- Review the test results.
- Notify the patient of both normal and abnormal results.

Nurses are involved in test results for review and disbursement. Physicians may give the nursing staff the responsibility of calling all patients with normal test results to explain the results to the patient, or the physician may want to see all abnormal test results and give the nursing staff instructions on what to tell the patient to do.

If the clinic has testing capabilities on site, the nurse may have to coordinate testing for the acute care patient. For instance, if a patient comes in for symptoms of a cough, the physician may order lab and a chest x-ray. The nurse will then coordinate with the onsite lab and x-ray department to run those tests immediately. After the test results have been received, the nurse will then have the patient see the physician again for a diagnosis.

Reports from other ancillary services will have to be collated. If the patient was sent to physical therapy, the reports may return through the nursing staff. The nurse may have to determine a process flow for that paperwork.

Other diagnostic testing may be done in the practice that will require nursing intervention. Stress testing or other cardiac evaluation requires nurses to monitor and administer medications, for example. Flexible sigmoidoscopies or other gastrointestinal scopes require a nurse to position the patient, instruct them about the procedure beforehand, and possibly administer medications. Nurses are involved in the premedication of radiologic procedures, including magnetic resonance imaging (MRI) and others.

Some practices sell products to patients or have a retail outlet. This may include vitamins, cosmetic supplies, eyeglasses, medical supplies, or pharmaceuticals. Nursing staff should know how this process works and what their role is in engaging the patient to purchase these supplies.

====================*FAST FACTS in a NUTSHELL*

- Ancillary services provide supplementary care in a medical office and vary widely in their form.
- Nursing plays a key role in assisting the patient to understand and follow through with the supplementary care.

CARE MANAGEMENT

Care management is a broad term used to describe the process of managing the entire patient population assigned to one physician. Most often, it is found in primary care offices. However, in some specialty offices, care management is also a key role of the nursing staff. Care management includes managing chronic illnesses and preventive care by engaging patients further in their health care.

Determining the needs of the entire panel of patients your physician or practice serves is part of the care management process. Technology can assist the nurse to compile data, analyze the data, and find opportunities in which patients can be notified and engaged to obtain further care.

A component of managing the patient's care is coordinating it across many different health care providers. For instance, the patient may enter the hospital or be sent to a referring physician. The nurse may coordinate that hospital admission by sending orders, a medication list, and progress notes to the hospital so that treatment can be coordinated more completely. When the patient is discharged, the nurse may obtain reports about the hospital stay, including history and physical, medication list, and discharge summary so that the patient can be treated appropriately.

Likewise, when a patient is sent to a specialist, the nurse will need to gather information (i.e., medications, progress, and reason for referral) to send to the specialist. After the visit, the consult report can be obtained so that care can be coordinated with specialist care.

On the other hand, a nurse in the specialist office may have to coordinate care by obtaining information from the referring physician, hospitals, or diagnostic testing facilities prior to the physician visit. After the specialist visit, the nurse may have to coordinate surgery, treatment, or further diagnostic treatments, and assist in sending information back to the referring physician.

Patients need to become engaged in their health care and have a continuous relationship with their physician, both primary and specialty care. Care management can become more difficult in today's world since patients often determine their own need for specialist or hospital care. Engaging the patient to inform you about their "other" health care activities is very important to managing their entire care. The appropriate use of specialty care to supplement primary care services can lessen the complexity of the system for the patient. Patients who are included as part of the health care team can be more active in care discussions.

Nurses are playing a bigger role in the care management of patients. This entails caring for not only those patients who come into or call the physician's office, but also those who do not. Understanding who the entire population is and what their needs are is the first step in care management. It involves managing those patients who are high users of the system and who may have multiple chronic conditions more intensely. It is also providing care for those who feel they never need a physician. Nurses can become actively engaged with patients to provide preventive care to both chronic disease patients and those who are healthy.

FAST FACTS in a NUTSHELL

- Care management includes managing the entire patient population assigned to one physician.
- Nurses are playing a bigger role in each of these areas to provide care in the office setting and avoid more costly inpatient care.
- Services provided in a medical office vary widely, depending upon the specialty and location. Care provided in a medical office may be evaluation and management, procedures, ancillary services, or care management.

3

Payment for Services and the Nurse's Role

INTRODUCTION

Nurses who work in medical offices require an additional set of skills, and it is important to understand those requirements before proceeding to understanding the role of the medical office nurse. Areas such as billing, coding, and reimbursement are not typical nursing knowledge areas, but they are very important areas in the medical office. This chapter introduces billing, payment of services, and the nurse's role.

In this chapter, you will learn:

1. How services are paid for.
2. The nurse's role in billing.

PAYMENT FOR SERVICES

In order for any medical office to continue to provide services, payment must be collected. Even free clinics have to receive payment for services, although payment is often not from the patients they serve. For most clinics, one of the most common reimbursement or payment mechanisms is health insurance. Health insurance can be private insurance (Blue Cross, Aetna, Cigna, United Healthcare) or government-sponsored insurance (Medicare, Medicaid, Tricare). Other payment mechanisms are workers' compensation, liability (injury due to someone else or someone's property), or self-pay, in which the patient is responsible for the bill.

========================*FAST FACTS in a NUTSHELL*

Payment mechanisms for medical office services are:

- Private health insurance
- Government-sponsored insurance
- Workers' compensation or liability
- Self-pay

In order to bill for services a list of charges, sometimes referred to as a charge master, is created that itemizes charges for all the services the practice provides. Most insurance carriers require a Current Procedure Technology (CPT) and an International Statistical Classification of Diseases (ICD-9) code be tied to every service that is provided. Therefore, most medical offices set up their charge master related to the CPT code structure.

A CPT is a numeric code that identifies the type of service provided by the clinician. The codes are organized from 10000 to 99999. Each set of codes (10000–19999, 20000–29999, 30000–39999, etc.) is separated into a particular type of service. For instance, the 10000–19999 codes are for dermatology procedures, such as lesions and excisions; 20000–29999 codes are musculoskeletal services, such as fractures; 70000–79999 are for radiology codes; 80000–89999 are for laboratory codes; and so on, up to the 90000 codes.

As discussed in Chapter 2, one of the main services provided in a medical office is evaluation and management (E&M). The 90000 codes are considered E&M codes and are related to the provider's exam of the patient. With the 90000 codes, there are different types of E&M codes, and for each type there are several levels of complexity. For instance, the 99202 code is for a new patient with minimal complexity, whereas a 99205 code is for a new patient with high complexity. Likewise, a 99211 would be a simple established patient visit, whereas a 99215 would be a complicated established patient visit. Categories for E&M codes are new, established, in-office consults, hospital consults, hospital subsequent visits, hospital admissions, nursing home visits, and preventive care visits.

CPT has A codes, D codes, G codes, J codes, V codes, and others that are used for special purposes. Of particular interest to medical groups are the J codes, which are for medications administered in the office. Each medication has a different J code.

The other numeric codes in ICD-9 are tied to a disease process or symptom, and are usually a three- to five-digit number. They are broken into sections, such as infectious disease, neoplasms, respiratory, circulatory, musculoskeletal, mental, digestive, pregnancy, genitourinary, and more. The more digits identified, the more specific the code. For instance, diabetes is ICD-9 code 250. However, if you have the ICD-9 code 250.60, it would be diabetes with neurological manifestations, a more specific code.

═══*FAST FACTS in a NUTSHELL*

All services require the use of a/an:

- CPT code.
- ICD-9 code.

Following a patient visit, the provider determines the complexity of the visit and codes the visit using the CPT code for the service that she provided. She then determines the ICD-9 code that relates to the condition or disease the patient presents with. This may be one or several, depending upon the patient's condition. For instance, a patient may present with symptoms of a cold and also has hypertension. His blood pressure has risen due to the over-the-counter (OTC) medication that he has been taking; therefore, the physician has to deal with the cold and the hypertension, so he would code for both of these conditions.

Furthermore, each CPT code has to relate to an ICD-9 code. If a patient presents with back pain and in the process of examining the back the physician notes and removes a suspicious mole, the CPT E&M code for the back pain evaluation (99212–99215) must be tied to the

ICD-9 code for back pain, and the CPT code for the surgical procedure (11001–11999) must be tied to the ICD-9 code for the suspicious mole diagnosis.

CPT and ICD-9 coding involves nursing as well. If the nurse gives an injection, there is a CPT code for the administration of the injection and a J code for the medication itself. If she gives two injections, there is a CPT code for administration of multiple injections and two J codes, one for each medication. She must also tie the CPT code for the injection administration to the reason she gave the injection, the ICD-9 code or diagnosis. For instance, if she gives an antibiotic, she must tie the antibiotic J code to the reason she gave it, for instance, a sinus infection.

Another example of how nursing is involved in coding is nursing visits, which are low-complexity established patient visits (99211). These visits can be provided by the registered nurse (RN) in certain instances. For instance, in oncology, a patient presents for an injection but in questioning the patient, the nurse determines the patient is running a fever and has a sore throat. She does a full assessment and consults with the physician, who instructs her to collect a strep screen culture and give the patient a prescription for an antibiotic. The nurse then instructs the patient on those measures, performs the test, gives the prescription, and then administers the injection the patient initially came in for. Since the administration of the injection is also an E&M code, she can only bill for the E&M 99211 with the J code for the medication. This can get rather confusing since the rules are complex.

===*FAST FACTS in a NUTSHELL*

> When a nurse provides a service in a medical office, he must tie the CPT code for the service to the correct diagnosis, the ICD-9 code.

After the coding is completed by the provider and verified by the billing staff, a claim form is prepared by the billing office. If the patient has insurance, the claim form is sent to the insurance company. Most practices send their bills electronically through a clearinghouse that sorts and sends the claim form to the insurance company. The claim form is processed by the insurance company, and payment is sent to the practice, either by check or electronic means. Each insurance company has a contract with the practice, which includes a fee schedule that determines the amount of payment the practice will receive for each CPT billed. The insurance company pays as per the contract with the individual practice.

Another caveat to know about payment of services is determining the value of each CPT code. Each CPT code has a respective relative value unit (RVU) that signifies the physician input into that particular service. For instance, an RVU of 0.8 would require less physician input than an RVU of 3.5. Higher-level E&M codes (99214–99215) would have higher RVUs than lower E&M codes (99211–99213). E&M codes 90000–99999 have lower RVUs than many other CPT codes, especially surgery and procedure codes (10000–69999). Physician input into a surgical procedure is generally considered higher than just examining the patient.

The RVU value is often used to determine the charges the practice lists on the charge master. For instance, the practice could set up charges using the RVU value multiplied by a dollar amount or conversion factor. So an RVU value of 0.8 multiplied by a conversion factor of $80.00 would equal a charge of $64.00. This provides consistency in the charges. CPT codes would have charges based on the RVU, so lesser-value RVU CPT codes would have lesser-value charges and higher-value RVU CPT codes would have higher charges.

This same methodology is used by insurance companies to determine the fee schedule for the services rendered. Medicare publishes its conversion factor every year (usually between $30 and $40). Other insurance companies set up their fee schedules to be a certain percentage above the Medicare fee schedule for a certain year. Thus, medical practices are never paid the full charge for the service provided.

The bottom line is that payment in a medical office is different from going to the grocery store and paying for groceries. What is charged is rarely what is collected. The difference between what is charged and what the insurance carrier pays is the contractual write-off. It is expected because of the contract between the insurance carrier and the practice. You might question why the practice does not charge what it gets paid. The main reason is that all the different insurance companies, sometimes more than twenty-five different carriers, pay different rates. The practice makes the best guess at what to charge, and it should be more than the best payer.

===*FAST FACTS in a NUTSHELL*

- Each CPT has an RVU.
- RVUs are used to determine the physician input of any service.
- The RVU can be used to determine the charge master and the fees the insurance company pays for services.

If the practice has a contract with a particular insurance company, it is considered to be a participating provider. Sometimes the practice does not have a contract with a particular insurance company and may receive the total amount for that bill, or the insurance company may have a fee schedule for nonparticipating providers. Medicare has a fee schedule for participating providers and another one for nonparticipating providers. Other carriers such as workers' compensation or liability may not have a designated fee schedule, and this will be negotiated individually at the time of service. You, as a nurse, may encounter this situation while providing care to patients. The patient may be with an insurance company who is not participating with your physicians. The patient may be responsible for the entire bill in this case, and care should be taken to explain all of this to the patient prior to initiating services.

Once the claim has been processed by the insurance carrier, the patient is sent a bill for the remaining amount, or patient responsibility. If the patient does not have insurance, the patient receives the bill without the claim going to insurance. If the statement sent to the patient is not paid within a timely manner, the account faces possible collection activity. Sometimes practices give discounts to patients who do not have insurance and/or patients with large balances after insurance.

Understanding the payment for services is important for the new medical office nurse for several reasons. First, nursing provides services that need a CPT code for billing, such as injections, EKGs, IV therapy, procedure kits, supplies, or lab draws. Nursing may also convey orders for lab tests or testing and give referrals to ancillary providers, who will request the ICD 9 codes so that they can do accurate billing. Nurses may also provide nursing visits (99211) and will need to understand how and when to use the code appropriately. Experience is a good teacher; however, rules for billing change frequently. Education about coding should be taught by a billing person or others familiar with coding rules. Regular discussions with billing staff assist the medical office nurse in understanding and remaining up-to-date with billing rules. Often, a cheat sheet of most frequently-used codes may be helpful in making coding easier for the nurse.

Nursing also plays a key role in discussions with insurance companies regarding pre-authorization for services, diagnostic testing, and medications. Nursing staff are frequently responsible for understanding insurance company requirements and ensuring that surgical services are pre-authorized prior to the procedure being performed. This requires completion of a form and/or a phone conversation to determine if the insurance company will pay for the planned procedure, based on the CPT and ICD-9. If the procedure is not pre-authorized with the correct codes, the insurance company may refuse to pay for the services, and often does.

Diagnostic centers usually cannot perform the services that are ordered without an authorization number. It can also fall on the nursing staff to obtain insurance pre-authorization for these services and to pass this information along to the diagnostic facility. Nursing can also play a vital role in obtaining authorization regarding prescriptions of certain medications. The insurance company may request more diagnostic information before authorizing, and nursing staff is usually fielding those questions.

===FAST FACTS in a NUTSHELL

Medical office nurses play a key role in ensuring that billing is accurate and complete by:

- Making sure nursing CPT and ICD-9 coding is correct and tied together appropriately
- Conveying orders for diagnostic testing
- Keeping informed since coding and billing rules change frequently
- Pre-authorizing procedures, diagnostic testing, and medications

Correct billing and coding is very important to the practice since reimbursement for services is tied to the ability of the practice to remain open. If incorrect or incomplete coding is given, the insurance company may reject the claim and the practice will not be paid for the services. For instance, an injection for a certain medication is covered for a certain ICD-9 code. The nurse provides the incorrect ICD-9 code and the claim is rejected. Or, a lab test is drawn, the wrong diagnosis is supplied, and the claim is rejected. The billing staff is required to research and correct the claim, causing much time spent on rework. If the nursing staff would have coded correctly the first time, the claim would have been paid correctly the first time.

═══════════════════════*FAST FACTS in a NUTSHELL*

- Understanding how services are paid assists the nurse to more fully understand her role in coding for services.
- Nursing has to keep updated on billing rules in a medical office, and this is a different, often unfamiliar, area of knowledge for nurses.

4

The Medical Office as Part of the Continuum

INTRODUCTION

Within the last fifty years, there has been a shift in the provision of care from inpatient high cost settings to outpatient ambulatory settings. Part of this is due to the public's demand for more convenient, high-quality care, and part is due to the growth of managed care in the 1980s with a focus on reducing the cost of care. Changing the reimbursement methods has reduced the amount of care provided in hospitals and increased the amount of care provided in ambulatory care centers.

In this chapter, you will learn:

1. How ambulatory care fits into the overall health care picture.
2. The role of the medical office in ambulatory care.

THE ROLE OF AMBULATORY CARE

Ambulatory care is provided to patients that are not inpatients of a facility where the care is provided. There are two different types of ambulatory care: hospital-based and community-based. Examples of hospital-based ambulatory care include radiology, laboratory, surgery, therapy (i.e., speech, occupational, and physical), and education. Hospital-based ambulatory care could also include emergency room care. Community-based outpatient services would include physician office settings, ambulatory surgery centers, urgent care centers, occupational health clinics, cancer treatment centers, renal dialysis centers, rehabilitation centers, psychiatric care services, and other community-supported services, such as public health departments or neighborhood health clinics. Home health and hospice programs are another form of ambulatory care.

Ambulatory settings will provide a combination of preventive, diagnostic, and therapeutic services with benefits of decreased cost and convenience for the patient. Often, this type of care is provided in lieu of inpatient care.

═══════════════════════════*FAST FACTS in a NUTSHELL*

Ambulatory care settings include hospital-based and community-based services providing preventive, diagnostic, and therapeutic services.

Many ambulatory centers provide preventive health services, with the goal of maintaining health and preventing illness. Evidence-based clinical guidelines are available for guidance with prevention. For example, mammography, colonoscopies, Pap smears, and other preventive tests ensure appropriate warning of cancer. Childhood immunizations prevent many childhood illnesses, and adult immunizations, such as influenza and pneumonia vaccines, reduce the spread of disease. Education on lifestyle risks help prevent further illnesses or injuries; examples include smoking cessation, obesity evaluation and treatment, use of seatbelts, child safety devices, and environmental safety teaching. This education enables the patient to be an active consumer and therefore become healthier.

Likewise, many ambulatory care centers provide diagnostic and therapeutic services. Diagnostic services include laboratory and radiology testing. Therapeutic services include treatment and rehabilitation from illness and injuries.

Because ambulatory care is a large part of the health care system, ambulatory care providers are one of the primary sites where patients receive their care. To reduce cost, overall management of a patient's chronic illness can be provided in the outpatient setting, with exacerbations of the chronic illness often needing inpatient care. Treatment of acute care needs, such as urinary tract infections, back pain, and flulike symptoms, can be managed fairly easily in a physician's office. When they are managed in the emergency room, the costs are much higher.

COLLABORATION WITH INPATIENT CARE

Inpatient care is necessary at times in treating of the patient's chronic care exacerbation, critical illnesses, or injuries. Collaboration between ambulatory and inpatient care will provide more comprehensive care. The surgeon's office needs to access the hospital record for past surgeries to determine how and when to provide treatment for current illnesses. The oncologist will need to collaborate with the hospital to manage the cancer patient's medications after dismissal, and the primary care physician will want to understand what happened in the hospital setting for his chronic disease patients so he can better manage them in the outpatient setting and prevent further hospitalizations. The continuum of care requires communication and collaboration among health care providers so that the best care possible can be provided.

═══════════════════════════*FAST FACTS in a NUTSHELL*

- Inpatient care is necessary to treat critical injuries and illnesses.
- Communication is vital so ambulatory care providers can continue with the treatment plan.

COLLABORATION WITH LONG-TERM CARE

Under certain circumstances, patients may require long-term care. Usually, the patient is unable to continue to care for themselves and needs the assistance of full-time residential or intermittent nursing care to maintain health. In much the same way as inpatient care, ambulatory care providers will need to collaborate with these health care providers to further understand their patient's needs. Nursing homes, assisted living facilities, in-home care, home health, and hospice programs provide long-term care services.

Long-term care providers send information with the patient to the ambulatory care office for use in caring for the patient. The information may need to be clarified with a phone call, since the patient may not be able to give an adequate history. Home health and hospice nurses can provide an extension of the physician's care by evaluating and treating the patient in the home setting. The physician may also make visits to the patient in the nursing home or home setting to further understand and treat the patient.

════════════════════════*FAST FACTS in a NUTSHELL*

- Long-term care is necessary at times when patients need assistance with full-time residential care or intermittent nursing care.
- Communication with these providers is needed to more fully manage the patient's condition.

THE ROLE OF THE MEDICAL OFFICE

Medical offices can provide a variety of preventive, diagnostic, and therapeutic interventions for patients. The variety is limitless, and many variations exist in both hospitals and privately owned medical offices.

The medical office is most often at the center of all this care, coordinating and collaborating with all of the players. The patients often return to the medical office to have their health care managed. For instance, the patient is in the hospital and is told to return to their primary care provider after hospitalization to resume care. Likewise, the cancer patient is sent back to the oncology office to resume care after receiving radiation. The medical office has the task of coordinating care across the continuum and assisting patients in understanding the total health care picture.

As a medical office nurse, you will touch many other health care entities, both in ambulatory and inpatient settings. Understanding how the system works in your community will assist you in guiding the patient through the maze. Often, it can be confusing and complicated for you, even with a health care background; think how much more confusing and complicated it is for the patient.

FAST FACTS in a NUTSHELL

The medical office is at the center of all care coordinating with other health care entities.

ESTABLISHING RELATIONSHIPS

Because of the need to obtain information throughout the course of treatment when patients move in and out of other settings, the ability to establish and maintain relationships among healthcare entities and agencies is important. Obtaining and using information can reduce duplication and provide a more comprehensive care system. Medical office nurses are often responsible for establishing relationships with other health care entities and with patients.

Patient engagement is also about establishing a relationship, and this is one of the most important relationships you as a nurse will establish. Teaching health promotion and disease management strategies requires behavioral change by assisting patients to identify and cope with the emotional demands of the illness. A continuous relationship with a physician and nurse can engage the patient in changing and realizing a healthier lifestyle. Sustained caring relationships change behavior. Patients need to be active participants in their care, planning, and goal setting. Self-management abilities need to be taught and supported throughout every encounter to improve patient outcomes.

This is the main challenge for you as a medical office nurse. Through your actions and relationships with patients, you have the ability to change the outcomes of the patients you touch. Because of the often long-term relationships you establish with your patients, you can have a huge impact on them and their health care.

=== *FAST FACTS in a NUTSHELL*

- Ambulatory care is an important and growing part of the health care picture, providing preventive, diagnostic and therapeutic services.
- Both inpatient and long-term care is needed throughout the patient's life span.
- The medical office is in the center of care and needs to collaborate with all to provide more comprehensive care.

5

The Role of Technology

INTRODUCTION

Technology is a great way to maximize the nurse's time and, if used effectively, can be a big part of patient care. Understanding the pieces of technology used in the medical office can help the nurse to use them to the greatest efficiency and to maximize resources for care. Nurses will need to understand how technology works in their practice.

In this chapter, you will learn:

1. The various technology components used in a medical office.
2. How each component affects nursing.

THE PRACTICE MANAGEMENT SYSTEM

A practice management system is used in every practice for scheduling, billing, and reporting. Many different types of practice management systems exist on the market, and each one has various features and functions.

Practice management systems can be independent or a part of an EMR system. If they are separate, there is usually an interface between the two systems to transfer data from one to the other.

The scheduling function of the practice management system allows appointments to be scheduled. This is accompanied by a data-gathering provision so that all information needed for the appointment will be collected at the time of the appointment scheduling. Pertinent information includes name, address, telephone number, date of birth, insurance carrier, and the reason for the appointment. Many other pieces can be collected at the time of check-in at the practice. The system will number the patient according to parameters set up in the system. Typically, the first patient is "1" and then sequentially numbered with each subsequent patient entered into the system. The appointment schedule usually is equipped to handle numerous appointment types and providers. There is usually a function that allows for scheduling into rooms and/or procedures.

Other scheduling functions may include scheduling for various locations, searching for future appointments, insurance referral tracking, and managing insurance information. As you are aware, patients often change insurance information during the course of their tenure with a physician. Most systems allow that information to be kept consecutively so that old claims will still be able to be worked along with new claims. There may also be an alert function with scheduling that allows billing or nursing to alert the front desk or anyone scheduling an appointment. The alerts might include billing issues, duplicate appointments, referral expirations, or any other important information.

================= *FAST FACTS in a NUTSHELL*

The scheduling function allows:

- Scheduling of appointments by provider, type, and location
- Data collection
- Insurance information management

The billing function ties to the scheduling function by creating a ticket number for every encounter or patient visit. This ticket number follows the patient through the encounter, the claim submission, and payment of the claim. It is an identification number that alerts the system that this patient had this encounter. Once the charge tickets are completed after the visit, either manually or electronically, the billing staff will then complete the ticket by ensuring that the ICD-9 and CPT code are supplied and the insurance information is present. They will then submit the claims on a regular basis (usually once daily) through an electronic clearinghouse through the practice management system. Most often, this is an electronic transaction, but could be paper-based if there is an independent payer or workers' compensation claim.

The claims are processed by the clearinghouse and sent back to the practice management system if any are incomplete. The billing staff will then investigate what is missing, add the missing parts, and then resend the claim through the clearinghouse. The clearinghouse sends the claim to the insurance carrier, who then decides to pay the claim or deny it. Once the claim is adjudicated (i.e., processed by the insurance company), a payment is sent to the practice. In addition, an explanation of benefits (EOB) is sent to the practice, often electronically through the clearinghouse. This is then downloaded to the practice management system and posted to the patient's account.

The practice management system records all billing transactions in the system so that a history is created, which helps the billing staff know what has occurred. Often, patients call because they do not understand their bill and an explanation is needed. The practice management system allows for a more thorough billing explanation.

Another billing function of most practice management systems is the ability to check eligibility of the listed insurance carrier. This can be done electronically by sending a batch of insurance numbers to the clearinghouse to verify the presence of insurance and benefits. This allows the front office staff to clarify any insurance issues with the patient when they check into the practice and avoid waiting until the claim is rejected or denied by the insurance company. For surgical practices or those practices that do high-dollar procedures, knowing whether the patient has insurance and what their benefits are can initiate discussions with the billing office prior to a large bill accumulating.

Another billing function is the ability to create patient statements, either in-house or by sending them to an out-sourced company. The patient statement typically lists all the transactions for each visit, which is drawn from the billing features of the practice management system. These typically can be pulled up in the practice management system so that billing staff can see what the patient is looking at when they call into the practice.

FAST FACTS in a NUTSHELL

The billing function of the practice management system allows for:

- Creation of a billing ticket
- Claims submission
- Claims adjudication
- History of billing transactions
- Eligibility checks
- Creation of patient statements

Reporting is a big function of any practice management system. This can include financial, billing, and schedule tracking. Most practice managers provide production numbers to physicians at the end of the month that can be produced through the practice management system. Reporting allows for the ability to track trends in coding, appointment scheduling, no-shows, appointment types, visits, accounts receivable (i.e., that which is still owed to the practice), charges, payments, adjustments taken, and write-offs, among others.

You will use the practice management system often to look at scheduling and to determine needs for the day. If you are responsible for any pre-authorization for procedures, the practice management system is where you will find information regarding insurance. You may also be involved in using the reporting function if you work with outcomes or care management.

ELECTRONIC MEDICAL RECORD

The EMR is replacing paper records in many practices. This is the clinical portion of the record: the progress of the patient, the medication listing, diagnostic testing results, and many more clinical aspects. The EMR provides accessibility to the patient record from anywhere in and, often, outside the office. The record can be pulled without having to get up and find a paper chart. EMRs have been praised as increasing the efficiency of office staff and providers; however, it cannot be just an automated paper record. Some workflow processes will have to be redesigned to make it as efficient as possible.

Various functions of the EMR include an electronic problem list (i.e., patient diagnoses and problems), medication lists, and clinical notes. Nurses will most often start the documentation of the visit in the clinical record with the vital signs and medication reconciliation. Evidence-based reminders may also be part of the nurse's responsibility, and can include preventive screening (i.e., mammography, colonoscopy, immunizations) and chronic disease screening (i.e., for people with diabetes, this would include a foot exam, eye exam, and lab testing). A checklist for depression screening, smoking cessation, or past social and medical history may also be the responsibility of the nurse. Sometimes the physician also wants the nursing staff to start portions of the history taking, such as chief complaint, history of present illness, and family and social history.

Electronic prescription writing is often a part of EMRs, which creates efficiency for prescription refills. Protocols can be created to allow the nursing staff to perform a good portion of refills. Messaging is also a big part of EMRs. The ability to send a message to the nursing staff instead of calling creates efficiency. Sometimes the nursing staff can be the communication vehicle to triage those messages so that the provider gets only those messages that require her attention. If patient education is embedded within the EMR, simply printing out relevant information can replace searching for a handout to give the patient.

Pre-visit planning is much easier with an EMR since the record can be reviewed at any time prior to the appointment without having to get the chart. Notes or reminders can then be sent to the front desk for pre-work before the visit, or necessary reports can be gathered prior to the appointment to further streamline the visit with the provider.

Most systems have the capability to interact with diagnostic testing facilities so that the results will be sent automatically to the physician's inbox for review instead of having printed lab results to collate. Some systems have the capability of creating a letter from those results to be printed and sent to the patient. A hospital interface allows information to flow between the hospital and the office for patients dismissed or admitted. The ability to quickly obtain an emergency room (ER) report, for example, can save the physician time and change the outcome of her decisions. Some bigger systems integrate all providers in one system so that consulting visit reports can be reviewed and the patient's care can be well coordinated.

Since the EMR is the main tool for recording clinical information, your role as a medical office nurse may often require you to use this technology.

FAST FACTS in a NUTSHELL

The EMR adds:

- Electronic clinical record
- Accessibility from many places
- Use of evidence-based guidelines within the record
- Checklists
- E-prescribing
- Pre-visit planning
- Messaging among team members
- Capability to interact with diagnostic testing and hospitals

PRACTICE WEBSITE

Another technology area is the practice website, which can have a huge impact on the practice and the ability to inform patients of office hours, provide patient education, and allow patients to get to know the practice prior to seeing a provider for the first time. A patient portal, which can be embedded into the website, can facilitate communication between the patients and the practice through the use of e-mails, appointment scheduling, prescription refill requests, insurance referral requests, or patient satisfaction surveys.

More sophisticated patient portals allow for electronic physician visits in a structured manner so that the provider may charge for simple consultations instead of the patient coming to the practice. For instance, a patient may have frequent urinary tract infections and be familiar with her symptoms and past treatments. She could initiate an electronic visit by recording her symptoms and past treatments, which the physician could respond to as an electronic consult.

Portals can also be used for communicating test results back to the patient. The test results can be added to the website for patients' review, and a note from the physician can accompany the results to explain them to the patient. The integration of a personal health record can also provide the patient with assurance that his care is coordinated with other providers.

Portals usually offer the patient a login to obtain their information and/or communicate to the practice. Those practices that have incorporated a portal into their practice website have demonstrated an increased patient satisfaction in the ability to access their physician. The patient's ability to communicate with the physician whenever they desire has improved access to a new level. Some practices expressed concern about older patients not having Internet capabilities, but this concern has been unfounded for the most part.

≡FAST FACTS in a NUTSHELL

A practice website can allow the patient to:

- Become informed about the practice
- Communicate electronically with regard to appointment scheduling, e-mails, prescription refill requests, insurance referrals, and patient satisfaction surveys
- Obtain test results
- Integrate their personal health record

REGISTRIES

Registries allow the practice to gather, collate, and report data into a usable format so clinicians can determine plans for care management. Registries take data from many different systems in the forms of claims data, testing results, pharmacy data, EMR, practice management data, and other formats and combine them into one report. This allows the end user to review a comprehensive report to determine care opportunities in both preventive care and chronic disease management. The registry can be part of the EMR or a separate system.

OTHER TECHNOLOGIES

Other technologies can be used throughout the practice and offer efficiencies to patients, providers, and staff. A kiosk at the front desk so patients can check themselves in can make the front desk more efficient and eliminate a waiting line at check-in. The use of a fax server to create an electronic form of all incoming faxes instead of printing on paper can create efficiencies for everyone and reduce the need for someone to sort and catalog those faxes. The fax server can then be managed and test results, hospital reports, consults, and other faxes can just be routed to the person or physician who needs to see those items. After review, the report can be signed off and remain a part of the record.

Credit card processing occurs in most practices at the front desk, but can also be offered at multiple locations through a website. Electronic banking is emerging in medical offices and used for its ability to provide access to online banking reports, scanning for automatic deposit of checks, and online bill payment.

A copy machine can be one of the most complicated pieces of electronic equipment in the office, with sorting, scanning, faxing, and printing functions. It also provides a way to give patients copies of any documents. This may be a very important piece of equipment to you.

One piece of technology that is used frequently in a medical office is the phone, and understanding the various features and functions is imperative for success as a medical office nurse. Specific useful functions include voice messaging, transferring, and others. As a medical office nurse, you will interact frequently using the phone system.

The dictation system is another piece of technology. The system may be a separate structure, portable tape recording device, or a phone number to call into. Although nurses don't usually use the dictation system, it is important to understand how the system works and how to get information from it if physicians dictate progress notes.

Other health system portals may be used by the nurse who is gathering information for the patient visit. These can include hospital and diagnostic testing portals to access information for patients. You may have a separate password and login for each portal and hospital system.

Understanding how to use each piece of technology and using it efficiently is often a challenge for nurses. If you find this to be true, ask for assistance. Your efficiency is important, and as you learn to use the technology correctly, your efficiency will increase. Technology itself does not make the office more efficient, but if used appropriately, it can create efficiency.

=====*FAST FACTS in a NUTSHELL*

- Key technology components, such as the practice management system, copy machine, phone, and credit card processing capability, are standard in most medical offices.
- More advanced technology includes EMR, a website with a portal, check-in kiosks, and registries.
- Nurses must understand and use technology to improve their efficiency.

6

Roles in a Medical Office

INTRODUCTION

Many players are needed to make the medical office function effectively, and knowing these roles will assist the medical office nurse. In hospital nursing, much is done in the background that never touches the clinical area. Medical offices are different in this respect because nursing often interacts with other staff. They might encounter questions from billing or help direct the front office. Nurses closely work with the providers and therefore require knowledge of these various roles.

In this chapter, you will learn:

1. The various roles of staff in a medical office.
2. How nursing relates to those roles.

PHYSICIANS

The most significant role of the physician in a practice is to see patients and generate revenue. Most of the practice revolves around this role, since physicians may often be the only revenue-generating source of the practice. Therefore, physicians provide the bulk of services in the medical practice.

If the practice is independent, physicians usually own the practice. As a physician owner or partner in the practice, the physician provides guidance on the policies and procedures of the practice and its strategic vision. They make the rules instead of someone making the rules for them. Depending upon the size of the practice, there may be a physician board responsible for overall governing laws, with various physicians playing key roles in oversight. Some physicians are on track to become partners in the business. This usually occurs when they add a contribution to the corporation, usually by being a productive and accepted member of the team. Other physicians may not want to be partners in the corporation, or for various reasons are not asked to become partners. They will then have less authority in the day-to-day operations of the practice.

If the physicians are part of a bigger health system, through an integrated delivery system, for example, they may be employees just like you. Or they could be a part of the leadership structure of the larger system and, therefore, have an impact on overall policies.

Physicians are either paid a straight salary or are on a production basis. This has an impact on the practice and you, as a nurse, since the physician may have expectations on how many patients he needs to see on any given day. Understanding the motivation of the physician you work for is imperative in providing the best possible support for that physician.

Regardless of whether the physician is an owner or employee, she is a leader in the practice because of her knowledge and expertise. Often, the practice allows each physician to establish his own workflows and processes, as if they are an independent practitioner. The resulting autonomy has to be carefully managed to reduce chaos and prevent an increased workload for selected team members. Streamlining as many processes and workflows as possible will result in a smoother running practice.

═══════════════════════════*FAST FACTS in a NUTSHELL*

- Physicians provide a significant role in the practice, providing services and generating revenue.
- Understanding physician ownership and motivation will help the nurse better support the work of the physician.

RESIDENTS AND MEDICAL STUDENTS

Often, physicians in private practice are part of the training for prospective physicians, residents, and medical students. Depending upon their level of expertise and their year in school or residency, the resident or medical student will play different roles in the practice, as determined by the physician. Medical students can perform parts of the history-taking and exam, with the physician stepping in to assist with review and medical decision-making.

Residents may be able to see patients independently in the practice with minimal physician oversight.

Nurses assist in guiding and coordinating the patient flow and utilizing the resident or medical student. The nurse may be asked to assist the student or resident in learning the various software programs, the transcription system, the phones, or to locate the physician. Although it may add to your day, helping a medical student or resident learn what actually happens in a medical office will assist a future nurse in working with that particular provider.

MIDLEVEL PROVIDERS

Nurse practitioners and physician assistants can be used in a medical practice in various manners. The midlevel positions can perform the following functions:

- Evaluation and management of patients (same-day availability, routine follow-up)
- Phone triage support
- Surgery assistance
- Chronic disease management
- Education
- Health assessments
- Nursing home rounds
- Hospital visits
- Call responsibilities
- Oversight of clinics (anticoagulant, chemotherapy)

Discussion should occur with the midlevel provider with regard to supervision, what services the provider can and cannot provide in the practice, how they will be trained at the practice, and what protocols are required for them to provide services.

Nurses will need to understand the role of the midlevel provider, as it may affect their work. Knowing their workflow, independent preferences, and who makes decisions creates harmony for all. Nurses may need to help other office workers and providers in understanding how the midlevel provider fits into the practice.

FAST FACTS in a NUTSHELL

Nurse practitioners, one type of midlevel staff, can perform a variety of functions in the practice.

NURSES

Registered nurses (RNs) may be used for many functions, including phone management, patient flow, nursing procedures, patient education, medication management, supply management, and coordination of care. As a nurse in a medical office, your role will vary, depending on your specialty and the particular physician you work for. The following is a general description of the nurse's role in the practice and will be further explored in Chapter 8.

Phone management can take a significant amount of time for nurses in many practices, as handling and triaging of phone calls in large part involves nursing staff. Phone calls vary in length, complexity, and required follow-up work. Quantifying phone calls can assist in identifying both staffing and process needs. Reasons for phone calls vary, depending upon the specialty. Patients call the practice to ask questions about medications, treatments, test results, symptoms, and many other issues.

The term "phone triage" is often used when discussing phone management. This task is both clerical and clinical in nature. The receptionist answering the phone determines if the call relates to nursing. Nursing then determines the patient's need and plan of action—whether the patient can be managed over the phone or requires a visit.

Another significant role for nurses is patient flow: the overall movement of patients through the practice. Patient flow begins with the preparation of the chart—either electronic or paper. Basic chart prep is having the chart ready when the patient arrives. Chart preparation may be done when the patient arrives or several days before the patient arrives if testing is required. Good chart prep is essential for the physician to provide the most appropriate care to the patient.

Rooming patients is a major part of patient flow. The goal in most clinics is to keep the providers moving. The patient is brought to an exam room, where the nursing staff records a brief history, takes vital signs, and ensures testing and/or chart prep is completed. The nursing staff will also prep the patient for the exam, which may include asking them to undress, setting out supplies, or obtaining consents. The variation in how rooming patients is completed is dictated by the physician. Specialty physicians, such as ophthalmologists or podiatrists, are not as concerned about vital signs as primary care physicians are. How much nurses are involved to assist with history-taking is also practice- and physician-specific. Understanding physician preferences is crucial.

As the physician sees patients, the nursing staff may then be asked to provide assistance during a procedure or exam. Male physicians often want another female in the room for breast or pelvic exams. Procedures such as biopsies or excisions may require the assistance of nursing staff.

Another nursing function is managing pharmaceutical representatives (i.e., drug reps) wanting to visit with the physician during office hours. Physician preferences vary on this issue, depending upon the need for samples. This is handled differently across the spectrum. Some offices have chosen to limit or deny access of pharmaceutical reps.

Nurses are usually responsible for physician orders and follow-up after the physician visits. If no orders are given, the patient may leave. Depending upon the practice, nursing or the physician may dismiss the patient. The last part of patient flow is getting the patient out of the practice or back to the front desk.

FAST FACTS in a NUTSHELL

Patient flow includes chart prep, rooming patients, providing assistance to the physician as needed, managing pharmaceutical representatives, and carrying out physician orders.

Nursing procedures performed on any given day may include medication administration; wound or dressing care; staple or suture removal; irrigations; testing procedures, such as EKG, spirometry, and vital signs; and lab testing, such as urinalysis, Hemoccult stool, glucose monitoring, or others.

Patient education before, during, and after the physician visit will be provided by both physician and nursing staff. Sometimes, education supplements that of the physician, and sometimes the physician will turn over certain education pieces. If it is done well at the time of the visit, patient education will reduce phone calls after the visit. Patient education, done poorly or incompletely, will either increase phone volume or cause you to lose patients. Education is the primary objective to any office visit in helping the patient understand and be an active participant of his or her care, even during a procedure.

Medication management is a large part of the nursing role in a medical practice. Nurses reconcile medications to update the medical record with each visit or phone call. They frequently assess patients for compliance with the medication regimen and side effects from such a regimen. Nurses provide medication administration in many forms: oral, injection, intravenous, epidural, inhaled. Sometimes narcotics are provided by the physician's office, and the nursing staff is responsible for administering, tracking, and stocking those medications. Nurses can play a role with prescription refills, too, depending upon a given protocol. At the very least, they field calls regarding prescription refills.

Nurses usually are assisting patients with samples, if the practice provides samples. They will also assist patients in finding indigent medication funding as needed. Medication teaching may also be done by nursing staff.

=======================*FAST FACTS in a NUTSHELL*

- Nursing procedures can include administration of medications, wound care, and testing procedures.
- Nursing patient education supplements physician patient education.
- Medication management is an important responsibility of the nurse.

Supply management is usually under the control of the nursing staff in maintaining, stocking, and rotating medical supplies and medications. Each exam room needs to be stocked with just enough supplies to ensure that at any given time the provider or nurse doesn't run short. Nurses are also challenged to not overstock each room and to keep enough supplies on hand in the supply closet. Typical supplies used in a medical office include dressings, needles, syringes and sutures, among others. Medications need to be checked for expired dates on a regular basis, and an ordering system is necessary to ensure that required medications are kept in stock. Nurses are also responsible for the supply of prescription pads, if used, and educational resources such as patient handbooks. Some offices keep some self-management tools on site, such as glucose meters, or orthotic supplies, such as splints, crutches, and casting material. Ophthalmology offices may keep contact lenses or eyeglasses in stock.

========================*FAST FACTS in a NUTSHELL*

> Supply management includes management of medications, medical supplies, and educational tools by stocking, rotating, and ordering.

Another area that nurses are usually responsible for is coordination of care between other health care entities, such as setting up durable medical equipment (DME), home health, hospice, or other community resources requiring orders from the physician. The maze of health care is often confusing to us health care providers. It is more so for the patient. The nurse can be, and usually is, a sounding board when patients become confused with the system. In addition, speaking with family members involved in the care of the patient can take up a nurse's time.

Hospital and nursing home admissions usually require physician orders, and nursing conveys these orders. Specialist coordination will require information to be coordinated between several offices, and nursing will initiate this contact as well. Nursing will also ensure that the patient has followed up with the respective specialist and that the consult report has been received. Any test ordered by the physician should be tracked to ensure that the result is given to the patient. Nursing can confirm that the patient is notified of both normal and abnormal testing results.

Insurance companies and third-party payers often require pre-authorization or case management, and this can be the responsibility of the nursing staff. Coding for pre-authorization, diagnostic testing, and nursing procedures that are performed in the office setting is also the responsibility of the nurse.

Care management functions include organization and collection of data, data mining, reporting and analysis of data, decision-making regarding patients who need follow-up or interventions, and performing interventions such as letters or phone calls. For chronic disease patients, these phone calls could include a large portion of patient education and teaching.

Patient engagement activities are part of the nursing role, as patients usually have a trusted relationship with their nurse. As mentioned, this could include being a sounding board, assisting the patient with education, or developing the relationship to foster a change in behavior with a noncompliant patient.

Other tasks, such as completing paperwork for The Family or Medical Leave Act (FMLA) or disability for the patient, are the nurse's responsibility. As you can see, nursing seems to be the catch-all for many supportive functions of the patient's visit.

A licensed practical nurse (LPN) can often be used in the same manner as an RN, with appropriate oversight. Depending upon the experience and skills of the LPN, the tasks they can complete may be almost equivalent to that of the RN. Obviously, analysis of their abilities should be done prior to assignment of tasks.

================*FAST FACTS in a NUTSHELL*

Nurses have many roles in a medical office, including phone management, patient flow, nursing procedures, patient education, medication management, supply management, and coordination of care.

NONLICENSED NURSING STAFF

Many forms of nonlicensed staff may work in a medical practice. Anyone without a license is considered nonlicensed staff. This can include medical assistants, nursing assistants, surgical assistants, specially trained operating room technologists, ophthalmology assistants, and other trained or nontrained staff.

Nonlicensed nursing staff can be responsible for rooming patients, assisting physicians with procedures, diagnostic testing, preparing the patient for the physician's visit, supply management, room cleaning, and simple nursing procedures such as injections, vaccinations, wound care, and others.

As a medical office nurse, you may provide supervision to nonlicensed staff and work side by side in providing care to patients. Knowing what this person's knowledge base and competency is may reduce missteps and help in understanding their role in the practice.

==*FAST FACTS in a NUTSHELL*

Nonlicensed staff can be used to supplement the role of the RN in many ways.

ADMINISTRATIVE STAFF

There are two different administrative staffs in most medical offices: billing and front office. The front office staff is usually the least paid in the office. They have to face angry or impatient patients throughout the day and receive negative feedback from providers and nursing staff. Their job is tough. Often, they have minimal education or training, and are placed in the position with only on-the-job training.

Regardless of their background or education, the front office plays a key role in the functioning of the practice. They provide phone management by answering and directing the phones or taking messages. Phone management also includes scheduling and triaging patients. The front office also provides check-in and check-out functions. Examples of front office staff include receptionists, schedulers, referral coordinators, check-in and check-out staff, and phone attendants.

As a new nurse to the practice, you should take a day or more to sit at the front desk to understand this role.

Appreciating the front office staff's role and need to multi-task can result in your understanding this role better and may ultimately lead you to have a better working relationship with the front office staff.

Billing staff ensure that coding is correct, prepare the claims, work the denials, post the payments, and initiate billing to the patients. They work with accounts receivable to ensure that all money is collected. They will also work with patients with past due balances. You will interact with billing staff throughout the course of the patient's treatment to verify billing codes. There may also be some interaction when a patient wants to schedule a particular procedure but has a balance due on their account. Billing should also be used as a resource for you to remain updated on insurance company rules.

═══════════════════════════*FAST FACTS in a NUTSHELL*

Administrative staff that help support care provided in the medical office are the front office and billing staff.

ADMINISTRATION

Depending on the size of the practice, there may be an manager. There are varying levels of managers depending upon responsibilities, education, and experience. A manager who has on-the-job training with minimal education is usually called an office manager. A manager with advanced education who provides strategic direction and management is usually called an administrator. A chief executive officer or chief financial officer may be named in larger practices. There are many varying levels in between, and often all managers are referred to as practice managers. Although the name is not important to most managers, it may be quite insulting to call an administrator the office manager.

The qualifications and expectations are different with an office manager compared to the administrator. An administrator is responsible to the board of directors and may have a designated physician that he reports to on a regular basis. This role is focused on strategic vision, financial, human resource, and operations management. This person may supervise department heads or supervisors, who provide hands-on operation oversight. Office managers have fewer strategic responsibilities and are usually focused on the day-to-day operations of the clinic, such as staffing, scheduling, and billing functions. Practice managers can be anywhere in between office managers and administrators.

Practice managers may also be from outside the practice and work for a management service organization or hospital entity. They still supervise staff and report to the physicians, but they are members of a different organization. Depending upon the physicians and management organization, the manager's responsibilities may closely resemble that of an employed manager. Since the manager is employed by someone other than the physicians, there may be a disconnect between the manager and the physicians or staff.

The remaining structure and roles in the practice are highly dependent upon the size and needs of that particular practice. Department managers may include front office supervisor, clinical supervisor, and billing supervisor. If the practice is large enough, there may also be a human resource director, coding supervisor, urgent care manager, risk manager, and others.

RELATIONSHIP WITH SCHOOLS

One way a practice can assist in the training of physicians is by providing internships or externships to schools, such as medical schools. This can also be done for nurse practitioner and physician assistant schools to train future providers. Nursing schools may need training sites to learn community-based nursing, and medical assistant schools require an externship to be completed in an office setting prior to graduation. Billing schools, such as for coding specialists, also require training sites.

If the practice were to offer training to students, a readymade supply of possible recruits for future positions is available. Practice members, physicians, and administration are able to watch potential future job-seekers as they learn, and the practice can ultimately pick out the best and brightest.

═══════════════════════════*FAST FACTS in a NUTSHELL*

The practice can be a training site for potential future medical office staff.

TEAM-BASED CARE

Learning how to work together as a team can create efficiencies throughout the organization. Team-based care means that every team member understands their role and is maximizing their knowledge and training. Tasks that do not require the expertise of a team member can be delegated to those members providing support. For instance, rooming patients does not require the expertise of the physician or RN, so that task can be delegated to nonlicensed staff. Another example would be phone triage. Physician expertise is not usually required to triage patient concerns; an RN can triage those calls and ask for physician expertise when needed. Tasks such as stocking rooms and assisting simple procedures could be delegated to the medical assistant, whose training and knowledge can be maximized to provide good care.

To maximize the use of the team, each task should be analyzed for the complexity and abilities of those completing it. Each team member's abilities should be examined and understood by all. Matching abilities to tasks creates a highly functioning team.

All members of the team need to communicate on a regular basis to ensure everyone is functioning with the same set of information. Sometimes, daily huddles or quick meetings can facilitate an update to maximize the team's use. Regular department and staff meetings also support the team concept. Physicians can teach staff to better manage patients with regular communication, whereas nurses can facilitate more integrated care by communicating regularly with both nonlicensed and administrative staff.

═══════════════════════════*FAST FACTS in a NUTSHELL*

To maximize team-based care:

- Analyze each task and identify needed abilities.
- Match each team member's ability to a specific task.
- Communicate on a regular basis.
- Provide extra teaching as needed.

DELEGATION

As stated previously, the delegation of nursing tasks to non-licensed nursing staff may occur in a medical office. You should take special care to ensure delegation is done competently. But first, you must know the role of the person you are delegating to, and the skills and competencies of the nonlicensed staff. A job description is a good place to start in understanding a role. To delegate a task, you should spend sufficient time explaining and reviewing it. Having the task demonstrated back to you helps ensure the task has been fully understood. If the task is new to the nonlicensed staff, documentation of the delegated task should be completed and perhaps included in their personnel file for future reference.

An open line of communication should be provided for the person who has been delegated a new task. If, for any reason, he doesn't feel appropriately able to complete the task, he should feel comfortable with approaching you for further instruction. Following up with the nonlicensed staff to ensure the task was completed appropriately and without difficulty provides closure and continued evaluation of the delegation. If the task is a lengthy one, the progress should be evaluated on a regular basis until completion of the goal. Coaching may be needed to correct or encourage completion of a task that was delegated. Communicating what worked and what didn't will help improve the skills for future task delegation. Allowing the nonlicensed staff to provide input in improving and/or changing the task for the better allows them to be an active part of the team.

=== *FAST FACTS in a NUTSHELL*

To delegate responsibly:

- Understand the role of person you are delegating to.
- Explain and review the task.
- Maintain an open line of communication.

Continued

Continued

- Provide follow-up.
- Give coaching as needed.
- Evaluate the results.

CHALLENGES

A medical practice does face challenges in relation to roles. There may be some distrust between midlevel providers and physicians because of role definition. A physician may not understand the role of the nurse practitioner and therefore fail to use them appropriately. For instance, the physician may be overwhelmed with patients needing acute care but not understand the abilities of the nurse practitioner to see acute care patients for him. The nurse can step in to help the physician understand how the nurse practitioner may help. There may also be some misunderstanding regarding supervision of the nurse practitioner. Most states require physician supervision, and the practice may vary on how this is accomplished. Reconciling the state's regulation with the practice's policies will provide a basis for using the nurse practitioner to their full capacity.

There may be some challenges for physicians in understanding the role of the nurse as more than a handmaiden or personal assistant. Nurses are trained in the art of caring, while physicians are trained in the art of curing. Caring can be demonstrated in many ways, one of which is being competent in the nursing role. Physicians are not always aware of nursing abilities and how that translates to their role. A physician may feel he has to see and do everything related to patient care until he understands and appreciates the nurse's role in supplementing the care he provides. Using protocols to establish parameters and guidance for the nursing role may help the physician become more trusting and appreciative of the nurse's contribution to care. It may take a series of discussions to change behavior and provide full understanding if a provider was trained differently.

Another challenge is that other members of the team may think that nursing is shown favoritism because of the required close working relationship between physician and nurse. This can create animosity and a nonteam-like atmosphere that interferes with patient care. The nurse can take the lead on this problem by including the administrative staff in those relationships.

Taking the relationship beyond a professional one can also be a challenge for others in the office. Nurse and physician relationships can and do stay on a professional level if the effort is made. For instance, a nurse in one practice was babysitting and doing other personal tasks for the physician outside the office setting. This could easily have been allayed by the nurse remembering and stating to the physician that she works for this person in a professional manner, not personal. A subtle message can be sent to the physician and to others in the practice, by using "Doctor" instead of first names. The physician should be called "Doctor" at all times while working in the office setting. Some nurses feel a sense of power when the physician allows them to call them by first name. However, this can be seen to cross the line between professional and personal.

═══════════════════════════*FAST FACTS in a NUTSHELL*

Maintaining professionalism in the office setting begins with addressing all physicians as "Doctor."

Other challenges in the office setting related to roles may be the physician leadership role. Regardless of whether the physician wants to be a leader, he is a leader by his very position in the practice. People look up to him and imitate his actions, good or bad. Physicians may create chaos or a tough working environment for those around them. Or the physician may have other roles in addition to seeing patients, which can be challenging for the nurse.

One thing to keep in mind when working with physicians is that they are human. They have the same problems and issues that we all have. Their problems seem to be magnified because we put them on a pedestal and think they can do no wrong. They can do wrong, however, and most of them acknowledge they are human.

Understanding those challenges and taking an active role in providing clarification can assist other team members in realizing that a misperception has occurred. Discussions among different team members to clarify roles and tasks, as well as processes, can make the team work better together. Allowing the misperceptions to continue will damage the relationships within the team.

FAST FACTS in a NUTSHELL

- Each member of the team has a specific role in the practice.
- Working together as a team can provide greater efficiencies in care.
- Communication among team members facilitates teamwork.

7

Quality in a Medical Office

INTRODUCTION

In recent years, medical practice staff felt they were providing quality care if the patient returned to the practice to see the physician again. If the patient thought they were not receiving quality care, they found another physician. Today, quality in a medical office is related to the ability to prove that the care provided is based on good outcomes in the clinical area; overall health care; financial performance; reduction of errors; and satisfaction of providers, staff, and nursing, as well as the patient.

In this chapter, you will learn:

1. Outcomes that can be measured to determine quality of care provided.
2. Outcomes that have an impact beyond the care provided in the medical office.

CLINICAL OUTCOMES

Across the nation, in many different health care settings, there is a growing disparity among care provided and resources utilized to provide that care. Every newspaper or journal gives numerous accounts of variances in how treatment was provided for certain chronic conditions at different hospitals. Another thing often reported is the difference between regions of the country in dollars and utilization of services. There is a growing trend to identify and use consistent guidelines to reduce the disparities in care, utilization of services, and dollars spent, which ultimately provides a determination as to the quality of such care. Many insurance companies and government payers are now collecting and reporting clinical outcomes using claims data. Although measuring outcomes is the first step, there are numerous problems with the insurance company providing outcome data. First, the claims data is delayed until payment has been completed. Sometimes this can be months after care was provided. Second, claims data tends to not always be accurate. Consequently, there has been a move towards having the practice collect and analyze their own measures using real-time data and take actions where needed.

Evidence-based guidelines are the basis for any measurement of clinical outcomes. The National Quality Forum has been a leader in identifying and prioritizing this work by publishing a list of measures to follow. Ambulatory care standards address both preventive care (i.e., immunizations, medication management, prenatal care, smoking prevention, and cancer screening) and chronic disease (i.e., heart disease, diabetes, hypertension, obesity, bone/joint conditions, mental health, and asthma/respiratory illness).

FAST FACTS in a NUTSHELL

- Clinical outcomes can be used to measure quality.
- Evidence-based guidelines are the basis for clinical outcomes.

Primary care offices are an optimal setting to assess outcomes on preventive services. Patients typically have a physician they identify as their primary care physician. The primary care office can gather all preventive measures received by the patient, and with access to these outcomes, they can then guide the patient in prevention of illnesses and improve the overall health of the patient. Preventive measures that could be measured are immunizations and screenings. The number of patients over the age of 65 who receive an influenza vaccination yearly is a preventive quality measure. The same would be the case for childhood immunizations or Pneumovax for the elderly. Other measures often performed are cancer screenings, such as mammography, colonoscopy, Pap smears, bone density, and prenatal care. Screening for depression and smoking cessation is also considered preventive care.

Specialty offices often perform some of the above preventive measures but could also have specific measures to collect. For specialty clinics, clinical outcomes are tied to the specialty. For a surgeon's office, clinical outcomes would be tied to the evidence-based guidelines for surgical procedures, (i.e., number of infections, antibiotic prophylaxis, thromboembolitic prevention, prevention of infection in the central line, and others). For an ophthalmologist, clinical measures might include postoperative vision, complications within 30 days, diagnosis of primary open-angle glaucoma or age-related macular degeneration, or comprehensive exam before cataract surgery. Clinical outcomes can be measured with every specialty.

FAST FACTS in a NUTSHELL

Both primary and specialty offices can measure quality.

Identifying and capturing individual patient information is the first step in identifying prevention gaps for the patient. Many EMR records have the capability to identify those measures needed based on age and gender. An example of this would be a point of care reminder, a listing of preventive measures for the fifty-year-old female that pops up during the physician's visit, which might include mammography, colonoscopy, and influenza vaccination. Keeping track of all preventive measures in one place provides the physician with a more complete picture.

Chronic disease outcome measurement could also be done by the primary care provider. Although they may not provide all the services, primary care providers are a good collector of such information, since they are usually the connector of all care provided. An example would be a patient with diabetes for whom the dates as to when the patient sees the ophthalmologist for retinal exams, or a podiatrist for foot care, are collected. Collection and evaluation of the laboratory results is usually done by the primary care provider. Even though care is provided by several different health care entities, the conductor is the primary care physician.

The ability to determine the needs of a particular population and to manage that population is called population management, and it is used for both chronic and preventive care. For instance, if a report is run for all women over the age of fifty who haven't had a mammogram, the practice has then identified a population that needs mammograms and they can manage that population. In order to determine the needs of all the physician's patients, the data that is collected must be in a format that is easily reported. Most practices require the use of a registry, either within the EMR or as a separate program. The registry allows the collection of multiple disparate data sources and brings all the results into a useable report.

Population management allows the physician to more fully understand his population or panel of patients and provide proactive care in managing both their preventive needs and their chronic diseases. For instance, for the patient with diabetes, through the use of a registry, the physician can pull up a report that demonstrates the care opportunities for all patients with diabetes. She may have 50 out of 200 patients who have not had a hemoglobin A1C (HbA1c) in the last year. Evidence-based guidelines (EBG) for diabetes recommend a yearly HbA1c, and effective management of the person with diabetes is indicated by a value of less than 9. Therefore, the physician would want to review and possibly contact those fifty patients to have the appropriate testing done. The same physician may find that 20 of her 200 patients with diabetes have an HbA1c over 11. She can then empower the nurse to more closely manage those patients. The nurse might contact those patients and set up a regular weekly phone call to monitor their blood sugar log or, if warranted, bring a patient in for more frequent appointments.

By monitoring clinical outcomes for her population, the physician and nurse can become more in tune with how healthy their patients actually are, what needs they must fulfill to become healthier or maintain their current functioning, and what the physician and nurse's roles can be in managing their patients' care more completely.

FAST FACTS in a NUTSHELL

Measuring clinical outcomes can help the practice better manage their entire population of patients.

OVERALL HEALTHCARE OUTCOMES

The ultimate goal of managing clinical outcomes is to have better overall health care or efficiency outcomes for the health care system as a whole. By better managing people with diabetes in the office setting, the physician can possibly prevent a hospitalization or an emergency room visit. By managing the preventive clinical outcomes and ensuring influenza vaccinations are given to most of his patients, the physician may be able to prevent an outbreak of influenza in his community. By knowing what his childhood immunization rates are, the physician might be able to increase those numbers with an emphasis for all team members to encourage immunizations, thus preventing illness.

Activities by the medical office can improve overall health care outcomes. Better coordination of care for and management of patients with chronic illnesses can reduce the hospitalizations and rehospitalizations of these patients. By having a good system in place to follow up on all those patients dismissed from the hospital setting, the physician can better manage the patient post-hospitalization with better medication management and assessment of patient status. Those patients will be better managed when they are dismissed from the hospital, thus reducing the need to return to the hospital setting.

The use of generic medications most often can result in similar treatment outcomes and offer savings to the patient and the health care system. A physician has the power to reduce health care spending by not always prescribing the newest and most expensive medicine. Reducing or eliminating pharmaceutical representative visits in the medical office may reduce prescribing of the most recently released medication. Measuring the use of generic versus brand name medication can be an overall health care outcome.

Providing better access in the office setting may reduce the need to use the emergency room or urgent care centers. The patient who cannot get into the physician's office in a timely manner is more likely to use another method of care. Often, creating a better ability to see acute patients can provide continuity of care for the patient and reduce the overall cost to the system. Patients who do not see their primary care provider with acute care needs often are told to follow up with them after the urgent care or emergency room visit, thus increasing overall health care costs.

A good care management system can reduce overall health care expenditures by better managing those patients to reduce hospitalizations, reduce disease, and prevent illnesses.

=== *FAST FACTS in a NUTSHELL*

- Efficiency outcomes reduce the cost to the health care system.
- Activities in the medical office can improve overall health outcomes.

SATISFACTION OUTCOMES

Many variations are used to determine satisfaction in a medical office. Several types of satisfaction will be discussed in this section: physicians, staff, nursing, and patient satisfaction. Looking at each type gives the practice another piece related to the practice's quality. Most practices look at patient satisfaction as the only outcome that determines quality. However, this is just one outcome.

Physician satisfaction is evident to everyone in the office. Satisfaction is demonstrated in the following manners: spending quality time with patients; allowing for problems or crisis moments without becoming upset; a jovial, friendly manner; or being approachable. These are the doctors we all want to work for and with.

Many factors contribute to physician satisfaction based on both personal and professional causes. Satisfaction for anyone is the connection between the effort and the reward. Most physicians say they would just like to see patients. The effort to see patients is connected to the reward: treating and curing the patient. Most often, this is the reason they went into medicine—to provide care to patients.

However, physicians can become dissatisfied for personal and professional reasons, too. If the physician is unhappy, he may attempt to disguise or temper his feelings in a professional manner or by disengaging from the practice. But more often than not, it will affect his work with patients and staff, including you. Dissatisfied physicians are easy to spot and hear; they are the ones who tell everyone their dissatisfaction with life, treat staff and patients abruptly, throw things, or generally are not pleasant to be around. It is a tough situation; your reactions are important and may need to be tempered. At times, you may need the support of management to help resolve the physician's discontent. Sometimes, it may be as easy as providing assistance with administrative functions or eliminating some responsibilities that can be delegated. The dissatisfaction often can be fixed if brought to the forefront and explored further.

Staff satisfaction is also important to the functioning of the clinic, as staff members regularly interact among themselves and with patients. Staff satisfaction can be measured with a staff survey that asks various questions to solicit feedback. Sometimes just having the opportunity to voice concerns provides an elevated awareness and motivation for staff to be more satisfied. Management that is responsive to staff satisfaction usually report the results back to the staff and work towards an understanding that will bring mutual satisfaction to staff and management. No one wants to work in a practice where staff is unhappy. Understanding motivations and worries of staff can empower management to fix issues. As with physician satisfaction, most staff issues can be fixed if further explored.

Patient satisfaction can be measured at the time of the visit or with a survey outside the visit. Both will work; however, the survey outside of the visit may be more beneficial since it will capture those patients that are not coming in to see the physician and the reasons why. Satisfaction surveys should be tailored to capture information about the patient's experience in the practice, including scheduling, check-in, rooming, provider visit, check-out, and billing. The ability to access the practice for an appointment as well as for a phone call should also be addressed. Once the results are tabulated, the practice can determine areas of opportunity that may help improve the quality of care in the practice.

Looking at all the satisfaction results on a regular basis will show progress in changes or improvements made. Sharing all results with the appropriate staff can lead to changes just by providing awareness. Benchmarking against past results can be a satisfier in itself, especially if the staff has worked to improve the practice's satisfaction scores.

Both staff and patient satisfaction can be obtained using focus groups instead of surveys. The use of a good facilitator, tabulating and sharing results, and working towards improvement are key measures to consider.

═══════════════════════════════════*FAST FACTS in a NUTSHELL*

Satisfaction of patients, physicians, and staff is important in delivering and measuring quality care.

FINANCIAL OUTCOMES

Most people who work in a practice want it to be successful and stay in business. One financial outcome that is obvious to you, a staff member, is the practice's ability to pay staff salaries that are competitive with other similar work. The ability to offer incentives or bonuses to staff that assist in the practice's financial well-being is also a good financial outcome.

Another financial outcome is the ability of the practice to provide quality, cost-effective care. This can be multifaceted as the practice looks at all expenses and reduces those expenses as appropriate. It also includes the ability of the practice to collect money for the services provided. And while doing both of those, the practice maintains clinical and satisfaction outcomes at the highest level.

============================*FAST FACTS in a NUTSHELL*

Financial outcomes evaluate the financial viability of the practice and can be employee-, physician-, or practice-specific.

SAFETY

One outcome that is usually measured only when it does not occur is safety. We measure those incidents in which the patient or staff was not safe, such as a needle stick injury or a patient fall. Safety outcomes can be driven just as well as other outcomes. How do you provide a safe environment for the staff and patients?

Some measures that show safety is a priority are:

• Making sure staff has the right equipment and the equipment is in good working order
• Having the right supplies available and ready to use
• Understanding patient safety issues and how they relate to the individual patient, such as having non-slip rugs at the entryway
• Involving staff at every level to contribute thoughts and ideas and provide feedback on safety measures

Practices that are successful in making safety a priority communicate it regularly to staff and maintain its importance in day-to-day operations. Saying one thing and doing something else does not convey safety as a priority.

For instance, a practice that says patient safety is important but does not provide a safe work environment can not expect staff to believe patient safety is a priority. Patient safety should always be at the forefront of patient care.

ERROR PREVENTION

In order to prevent errors, everyone must know what potential errors could occur, what errors have occurred, and how to prevent a recurrence. Tracking errors by type, timing, and department can start this analysis. An environment in which errors are reported and openly discussed will lead to fewer errors as staff are taught safety measures for prevention. A reduction in errors may result as staff are better educated and aware of how to prevent further problems. Quality of care will improve as a result.

RISK MANAGEMENT

Risk management is the ability of the practice to reduce or eliminate any potential risks. Most practices have policies and procedures in place that identify and educate staff on proper processes. Often, these are guided by regulations. Such polices could include:

- Human resource guidelines
- Infection control
- Privacy and security
- Compliance plan

- Clinical protocols
- Billing procedures
- Handling of cash and monies in the practice
- Financial reporting

Regular and frequent staff education is one of the best ways to reduce risks in a medical practice and, therefore, increase the quality of care.

================================*FAST FACTS in a NUTSHELL*

- Quality can be measured by evaluating clinical outcomes, efficiency outcomes, satisfaction, and financial results.
- Safety and error prevention measures help ensure staff and patients can operate in a safe environment.
- Risk management education can be used to carry out regulations and teach staff the appropriate processes.

8

Maximizing Nursing's Role

INTRODUCTION

Once there is a clear understanding of the nurse's role, it is much easier to determine how that role can be maximized. This chapter explores nursing roles once again and takes a more in-depth look at how the nurse can work at the highest level possible.

In this chapter, you will learn:

1. The benefits of an RN and nurse practitioner in a medical office.
2. Operational efficiencies to be taken to maximize those roles.

DETERMINING THE RN ROLE IN THE OFFICE

It is sometimes difficult to determine the true need and benefit of having an RN in the medical office. Often, administration and physicians look at the bottom line and determine they cannot afford a registered nurse and thus make the decision to hire a nonlicensed nursing staff to carry out nursing tasks. Most of us would agree that it does not require an RN license to room a patient or stock rooms. And we might also agree that if the physician wants to handle everything in the office setting, from simple phone calls to patient education, that it is her right to do so. However, if an RN is a part of the team in a medical office, the physician might be able to see more patients, spend more time with patients, and provide the care that justifies the medical degree she spent many years obtaining.

There are many benefits of having an RN in the practice, and often these benefits are intangible, such as increased patient understanding of a treatment protocol or disease process, reduced risk of patient hospitalizations or rehospitalizations, improved reputation of the physician and office, reduced malpractice claims, reduced compliance and training costs, increased professionalism of the office, and improved work environment for the physician. Tangible benefits may be the increased ability for the physician to perform those functions and use the skills that she was educated to perform, instead of administrative and clinical oversight of nonprofessional staff. Another benefit is the ability within the office to have a true team caring for the patients, with each member supporting patient care and not always depending on the physician to provide all the care.

The RN role in the medical office should be thought of in the same manner as the physician's role in delegating tasks. If the RN is freed up to perform those tasks for which she went to nursing school—critical thinking, advocacy, patient education, and care coordination—the team functions at the highest level possible.

Nursing functions can be divided into the following categories:

- Facilitation of operations: ordering supplies, rooming patients
- Nursing procedures: medication administration, vital signs, diagnostic testing
- Nursing process: determining how best to assist patients through diseases, problem-solving concerns
- Telephone communication and triage
- Advocacy: working with patients to obtain better care
- Patient education
- Assisting with high-tech procedures: assisting and preparing patients for procedures, monitoring patients, post-op care, and follow-up
- Care coordination: coordinating care across many spectrums
- Quality improvement: care management of patient clinical outcomes

When you look at all the nursing tasks, some obviously could be delegated if taught and supervised appropriately. The following is a list of nursing tasks that could be performed by nonlicensed staff:

- Rooming patients, including chart prep, vital signs, history-taking
- Assisting the physician with simple procedures
- Diagnostic testing procedures: EKG, spirometry, waived lab testing

- Review of medication lists
- Acquiring samples
- Stocking rooms
- Supply management
- Insurance pre-authorization and follow-up
- Referrals to specialists
- Communicating with community resources
- Simple nursing procedures: removing sutures, dressing changes, etc.

More specialized and complicated tasks can also be delegated with intense training and competency validation. A nonlicensed staff person can assist with the following:

- Injections: allergy, subcutaneous, intramuscular (requires extensive teaching)
- Tuberculosis (TB) testing
- Vaccinations
- Wound care
- Medication refills
- Answering the phones and taking messages
- Simple patient education

======================*FAST FACTS in a NUTSHELL*

Nonlicensed staff can add value to the practice by supplementing the role of the nurse in various ways.

Because of the need for critical thinking and superior expertise, a licensed nurse is much better in certain situations. These include:

- Phone triage in which the nurse gives the patient advice or nursing care over the phone, reviews symptoms, or provides teaching
- Administration of chemotherapy, IV medications, or complex injections
- Care management and care coordination for complex patients
- More extensive patient education

Three factors should be considered when deciding what level of nursing care to provide in a medical office:

- What is the cost difference between the two options?
- What are the required tasks of the position?
- What outcomes do the physicians, administration, and other nursing staff want to achieve?

RNs can add value to the team in the form of better outcomes for the physician and the practice. Hiring an RN does increase the cost to the practice, but that cost can be mitigated by allowing the physician to perform other functions that might generate revenue to offset the cost difference. An example of this is a physician who typically spends one hour per day answering phone messages taken by the front office. In addition, she spends thirty minutes approving refills for patients.

After an RN is hired and takes on these two responsibilities, the physician can see four more patients in that same time, thereby generating revenue that offsets the cost of the RN.

═══════════════════════════*FAST FACTS in a NUTSHELL*

Making a decision about licensed versus nonlicensed staff comes down to cost, outcomes, and need.

DETERMINING THE NURSE PRACTITIONER ROLE IN THE OFFICE

Nurse practitioners are used in medical offices with increasing frequency, especially primary care practices, due to the growing shortage of physicians. Use in specialist offices has also increased. There are several options for using the nurse practitioner, and they vary widely by specialty. Options include:

• The nurse practitioner functions as a primary provider for patients, and patients establish their care with this provider. Patients may never see the physician or only occasionally as the need arises. Arrangements may be made for the physician to see the patient every third or fourth visit. This arrangement is seen more frequently in a primary care office.
• The nurse practitioner supplements the role of physician and collaborates with the physician to care for

a panel of patients. The nurse practitioner may see patients for follow-up or routine visits, assist with hospital or nursing home rounds, handle phone triage, and assist with call coverage, which in turn frees up the physician. The nurse practitioner does not have her own panel of patients. This arrangement is seen in primary care and most often in specialty offices.

Both options work well in many different environments, depending upon the practice structure and type of physician leadership. There is controversy between the use of physicians and nurse practitioners in some areas of the country, and this is usually related to a disagreement regarding scope of practice. In most cases, however, the nurse practitioner and physician can work quite effectively together in the office setting, especially if time is taken at the beginning to define the role expectations and clarify any misconceptions.

The benefits of having a nurse practitioner in the office are numerous and vary based on the role assumed by the nurse practitioner. Benefits may include the ability of the physician to maintain his panel of patients more effectively, spend extra time with chronic disease patients, and provide optimal hospital care. The nurse practitioner can usually spend more time with patients, provide a more comprehensive collaborative approach to patient care, offer more intense teaching or phone triage, and provide another resource for the staff and others.

====================== *FAST FACTS in a NUTSHELL*

Nurse practitioners can be used in various ways, and the practice will benefit from their services.

MAXIMIZING THE ROLE DEFINITION

One challenge for you as a medical office nurse is to have a thorough orientation when you begin your career in ambulatory care. Ambulatory care is not emphasized or explained fully at most nursing schools; therefore, the nurse usually finds herself without resources or experience to fully maximize her role. Medical offices can often hinder orientation since staff is usually needed for their regular duties, and the new orientee is put on the job with minimal training. Whether you have to formalize your orientation or it is provided for you, it is important to take some time initially to understand the office. Initial orientation in a medical office should highlight these areas:

- Organization of the medical office (i.e., structure, scheduling, staffing, culture, competencies, etc.)
- Roles of all staff members and how they relate to your position
- Policies, procedures, and protocols (both written and unwritten)
- Types of care provided in the office
- How triage works: assessment, disposition, and documentation

- Available decision-making resources
- Current communication between members of the team
- Quality outcomes
- Patient education resources
- Current collaboration among external and internal systems
- Technology applications and systems
- Reimbursement and any external regulations that apply to nursing

As you become better acquainted with your responsibilities, the office in general, and the above processes, you can then define how you fit into the practice. There may not be a set role for the RN, or even for the nurse practitioner. Each situation may be unique and require you to define your specific role. This may take some time, especially if the role is new to the practice. Even if the role is not new, there may be some preconceived ideas regarding what a nurse should do, and you will have to clarify and possibly re-educate those around you.

Understanding the roles of all team members is the first step in identifying your role as a medical office nurse. If there is a job description, it might give you some insight into what is possible. Numerous resources and organizations may also provide guidance. Ask your practice manager for these resources. Talking to other nurses in other medical offices can help to clarify your role. Having frequent discussions with the physician(s) will help clarify matters for all. Together, a clear role can be defined.

==*FAST FACTS in a NUTSHELL*

- Orientation is important to understand the role of the nurse.
- Defining your role in the practice will take time.

OPERATIONAL EFFICIENCY MEASURES

Many efficiencies can be implemented in the medical practice that will make your role more efficient. This section will expand the discussion in Chapter 6 regarding phone management, patient flow, nursing procedures, patient education, medication management, supply management, and the all-inclusive category of coordination of care.

Phone Management

In every practice there is a different method for handling nursing phone calls. In efficient offices, the phone call is taken by administrative staff, and a message is written either electronically or on paper and attached to the medical record. Information that may be useful in answering questions should be reviewed prior to answering the call. A brief review of past medical history, medications, and most recent visit documentation can give the nurse a quick overview of the patient's status. Nursing should be wary of answering phone calls without having the medical record to refer to, due to liability issues.

Determining who is responsible for phone triage is important. The use of the team is maximized if one person is responsible for triaging calls and obtaining physician intervention as necessary. In one practice, three nursing staff were responsible for messages for one physician. After taking the call, each nursing staff would try to find time to consult with the physician. This created a chaotic situation. If one nurse would have taken all messages, he could have consolidated his discussion with the one physician.

Nursing phone triage is the process in which the nurse, after discussing the patient's health situation with the patient, makes a determination as to the treatment protocol. This may involve one of the following patient care activities:

- Symptom assessment
- Counseling
- Home treatment advice
- Referral information
- Disease management
- Crisis intervention
- Physician referral
- Health information topics
- Appointment scheduling
- Authorization services

To effectively perform phone triage, certain skills are necessary. An efficient phone triage nurse will have the following characteristics:

- Excellent communication skills
- Critical thinking skills

- The ability to handle stressful situations
- The capacity to function independently
- Varied clinical experience, including hospital nursing
- Ability to document conversations and patient teaching

Phone triage requires the use of the nursing process— assessment, diagnosis, treatment, and evaluation. The nurse assesses the patient's concern and makes a nursing diagnosis, which is different from a medical diagnosis. A nursing diagnosis involves the assessment of subjective and objective data to form a conclusion as to the needed actions and then evaluating the results. An example would be the patient who calls in to report symptoms (objective data) and how they feel (subjective data). The nurse determines that the patient needs to be seen by a physician. In contrast, a medical diagnosis would be the physician taking an after-hours call from a patient reporting symptoms. The physician diagnoses the disease and prescribes medications over the phone.

Once the nursing diagnosis is made, treatment is given. This may be nursing advice, such as ice packs or rest, or consulting a physician and informing the patient of the prescribed treatment plan. It may also involve the decision to have the patient come into the office. The treatment may or may not include the physician. The final step is evaluation. With phone triage, this might involve having the patient reiterate the given instructions or voicing understanding. It may be instructing the patient when to call back if problems are unresolved, or it may be a follow-up phone call by the nurse several days later.

True nursing phone triage carries the risk of liability. An example of this is a mother of an infant who calls to report that her baby is crying constantly and telling the nurse she didn't think the baby was getting enough breast milk. The nurse advises the mother to start the child on rice cereal to supplement the breast milk. That evening, the infant is brought to the emergency department and diagnosed with meningitis, a serious condition that could lead to death. The nursing staff may have done everything correctly, or they may have missed a subtle clue indicating that the patient should have been seen.

To reduce the liability risk, nursing phone triage should be carefully considered. Well-designed procedures, staff competency verification, and documentation guidelines should be in place prior to implementation.

Procedures could include the following.

- Risk management (working with minors, angry callers, noncompliance, power failure back-up systems, nursing across state lines, etc.)
- Process (defining guidelines, calls that do not fit into a defined guideline, medications, lab testing, emergency calls, prioritizing calls, making referrals, etc.)
- Clinic issues (who receives the call, access to records, when is the patient seen, etc.)

Numerous resources are available to develop guidelines, or they can be created in-house. These should be evidence-based guidelines and follow nationally recognized standards of care. They can be symptom- or disease-based. A simple example may be a protocol for constipation. As we all know, there are simple measures to take before seeing the physician, and there are also warning signs of when the physician needs to be seen immediately for this complaint.

Staff competency is vital in making phone triage successful. The most important competency is licensure. Only RNs or experienced LPNs should attempt true phone triage. Phone triage requires critical thinking skills and a background in the nursing process. Experienced nurses make better decisions than new graduates because they have been exposed at one time or another to different situations during their career. A review of all phone calls and how they were handled by a supervising physician may be helpful in determining the abilities and knowledge base of the triage nurse. A continuous monitoring system should be implemented.

FAST FACTS in a NUTSHELL

- Phone triage is a main function of nurses in a medical office.
- Knowing the difference between phone management and phone triage is crucial before implementing a program.

Patient Flow

If chart prep is performed prior to the visit, the patient will be better prepared to see the physician. The nurse can review the last visit, gather any tests performed since the last visit, or provide guidance to the patient to bring films, medications, or other items to the appointment. Perhaps this is a task that could be delegated to a nonlicensed chart prep person who has a good understanding of diagnoses, testing, and how to think clinically about what may be needed for the visit.

Processes should be established so that the appropriate tests are on the chart prior to the follow-up appointment. How the test result moves through the practice is important to understand. Is it on the physician's desk awaiting signature? Is it held in a file awaiting the next visit? Is it filed immediately? Is it with the chart? All of this should be explored to ensure that an efficient means of routing is used and chart prep can be completed. Use of an EMR helps eliminate the endless search for results.

Rooming patients should be done quickly but thoroughly. If rooming patients seems to take a significant amount of time, each step in the process should be evaluated for efficiency. In one practice, several minutes were taken with each elderly patient helping them on and off of the scale. A simple suggestion, lowering the scales into the floor so that older patients had an easier time getting onto the scale, saved tremendous time.

One skill that is vital for good patient flow is the ability to make the patient comfortable, but at the same time keep the physician moving. In one instance, a physician had an assistant who was personable and loved to chat with patients and make them comfortable prior to the physician entering the room. However, the physician often sat and waited for the assistant to complete his "chat" with the patients. The assistant did not have the ability to "break away" from the patients and keep the physician moving. Nursing's role is to seek information from the patient in a quick and friendly manner.

The use of flags or lights could be helpful to streamline communication with the physician and show what is happening with the patient in any room (i.e., roomed and ready for the physician, lab needed, nursing follow-up needed, etc.). Anticipating the physician's needs can assist with patient flow. If the patient will need labs, radiology, or prescriptions, these can be placed on the front of the chart or prefilled in an electronic chart so the physician has ready access. Preprinted prescription pads for frequently used prescriptions also assist the physician to move faster since he only has to sign and hand them to the patient. Examples could include bowel prep or antinausea medications for oncology patients.

═══════════════════════════════*FAST FACTS in a NUTSHELL*

Patient flow includes the following functions:

- Chart prep
- Gathering the appropriate testing before the visit
- Rooming patients efficiently
- Making the patient comfortable
- Communicating with the physician

Nursing Procedures

Creating efficiency with regard to nursing procedures is related to where the procedure occurs and what supplies are needed. Most nursing procedures, such as dressing changes, suture removal, casting, or catheter irrigation, are carried out in the exam rooms after patients are seen by the physician. The room should be stocked for those procedures that occur frequently. However, it makes no sense to stock a room just in case you will apply a cast to a patient. Because of the cost and volume of casting supplies, a separate room should be set up. Think about all the nursing procedures that will be done in the room and then stock the room accordingly. A separate nursing procedure area may be created that could add efficiency and streamline tasks.

Patient Education

Patient education tools can be made more efficient by placement, content, and understanding of content. For an orthopedic office in which total knees, total hips, or arthroscopy are the main surgical procedures performed, a supply of those patient information handouts could be kept in the exam room. For a more varied general surgeon, there may be two dozen different procedures performed, and keeping related handouts in the room would not be efficient. A primary care office may find an electronic program that has a wide variety of topics to be more practical. Printing the right handout can be done at the time of the visit. Location of any education tools should be within easy reach of the exam room.

It might be cost-effective to develop these education tools if they are used frequently in your practice. If all the physicians perform hernia repairs, for example, and similar instructions are agreed upon, a nicely printed sheet or booklet could be prepared to give to patients. This may make patient education more efficient since it is tailored to your office. Some offices provide the patient with a care plan that includes medications, diagnosis, and patient education related to the visit.

The patient also could be directed to visit various Internet sites for information. A neatly printed handout will allow the patient to take the information home, or the patient could be directed to your website to link to resources. You could have preprinted handouts available for those who do not have Internet access, but you may find that a large percentage of patients want to do some exploring on their own, if they haven't already done so.

Even if you have prepared patient education tools, nursing staff needs to take the time to briefly explain the reading material. Make sure you have read and understand what you are teaching. Also make sure phone triage staff have read your patient education materials. Phone call volume will increase if handouts are not correct or are not explained fully.

═══════════════════════════*FAST FACTS in a NUTSHELL*

- Patient education should be located so that these items can be easily located.
- The more frequently used patient education tools should be tailored to your practice.
- Taking time to educate the patient will reduce phone call volume.

Medication Management

A good medication sheet will allow for clear identification of current medications the patient is taking, along with changes during the course of treatment. Primary care offices may want a more detailed listing since they usually follow the patient over several years.

With every visit, the nursing staff should ask about any changes in the patient's medications. This may be difficult for the patient to remember, so having the patient bring their medications may streamline this process. Some physicians want nursing to obtain a complete medication listing at the visit, while other physicians review medications with the patients. Samples, over-the-counter, and supplement medications should also be listed on the medication sheet.

When medications change, either at the office visit or with phone triage, the medication log should be updated. These logs are often used during subsequent phone triage, office visits, and/or admission to the hospital setting. Keeping an updated medication log is more efficient than leafing through ten pages of progress notes to find all medications. If the physician can assist with this, the medication record is more complete. And, of course, an electronic format will save time.

═══════════════════════════*FAST FACTS in a NUTSHELL*

- Medication management includes a good medication sheet to identify and track changes.
- Medication reconciliation should be done with each visit.

Efficiency in medication administration is limited to the type of supplies and their location. Medication administration cannot be hurried, but it can be made more efficient if supplies are readily available and user-friendly. Location of the supplies should be in close proximity to where they will be used. It is not efficient for nursing staff or physicians to have to walk clear across the clinic to obtain samples or medication for an injection. Medications should also be kept out of reach of patients, so storing them in exam rooms should be limited. Supplies that require a tremendous effort, such as Tubexes, should also be reduced. Nursing staff should know how to use supplies appropriately.

Patients should be kept in the office for an adequate time after an injection to ensure there is no adverse reaction. This will vary by medication, frequency of injection, and/or patient's history of taking the medication or past side effects. The patient can be asked to wait in the reception area for the given period with instructions to notify nursing when they are leaving and/or if there are any symptoms.

For many practices, the most frequent physician order given is for refills. Sometimes five different methods are used to refill medications for five different physicians. For instance, one physician may refill all prescriptions for one year, another for only three months. Although it will take some effort, the physicians and nursing staff who agree on how the process should be handled are more efficient. A procedure to establish the ground rules for refills could include the following guidelines:

• The dosage of the medication must match the medication log, physician's dictation, or a message contained in the chart.

- The patient is still under the physician's care and has not been dismissed from the practice.
- If the patient has not been seen within the prescribed time, a month's prescription will be given and the patient has to make another appointment.
- Generic medications are approved unless otherwise stated by the physician. If certain drugs should not be refilled in generic form, a list could be made.
- All patients have been seen within the last twelve months.
- Any medication not on the refill table has to be approved by the physician.
- The procedure and refill table is reviewed by the physicians yearly.
- One-year prescriptions can only be filled by the physician.
- Narcotics can only be refilled by the physician.

A refill table can be created to break down classifications of medications and establish guidelines for how often the patient needs to be seen in the office, how often lab needs to be done, and how many refills can be given.

In other practices, the physician may want to see every prescription refill request or designate a nurse practitioner to handle refill requests. A guideline or protocol should be established for the nurse practitioner as well so there is no misunderstanding between provider and physician. Nurse practitioner prescriptive authority varies from state to state, so you will want to be aware of your particular state's regulations. Refill requests and refill orders should be documented, either on the medication sheet or in the medical record.

A primary care practice can become inundated by refill requests. One thing that is helpful is for the patient to be told to call the pharmacy for refills. The physician's office only takes refill requests from the pharmacy. If the pharmacy faxes over refill requests, the fax machine should be located by medical records so that the record can be pulled to place with the refill. Using electronic prescribing (e-prescribing) to handle refills is a much easier process for the practice. There may still need to be a process for handling refill faxes from pharmacies or phone calls from patients, but sending an electronic prescription saves time on the phone. Most e-prescribing systems have checks and balances to ensure safe medication management.

One way to reduce phone calls for refills is to ask the patient about them at the appointment. This can even be included on the pre-visit sheet. Another option is to have a refill tablet or sign placed in the exam room that alerts the patient to ask for refills. If a tablet is used, the patient can tear off the sheet after writing down those refills she needs. If an EMR is used, nursing staff can review the need for refills and alert the physician as to which medications need refilling.

======================*FAST FACTS in a NUTSHELL*

- Medication refills will consume a large amount of time in any office, especially primary care.
- Protocols that have nursing provide support for medication refills will help streamline this process.

Supply Management

Stocking rooms regularly will save a lot of time while seeing patients. A regular stocking schedule could outline and identify what is needed. Most of us assume that everyone knows what and when to stock; however, this is not always the case. Reviewing and teaching stocking practices will save time in the future.

Developing a list of supplies that should be stocked in each room allows anyone to stock rooms during downtime. Stocking duties are usually delegated to nonlicensed staff and are often the last thing done. Stocking has to take priority and should be done on a consistent schedule each day to save time.

How the rooms are stocked and with what supplies depend upon what the physician uses at each visit. In some practices, physicians share rooms due to space considerations. If there is a chance that nursing staff or physicians may work in different exam rooms, each room should be stocked in a similar fashion. In any specialty practice, a physician can add an office at the last minute to accommodate patients when another physician is already using his regular rooms. Since common items are used at each visit, each room could have one container that sits on the counter. It includes the same items in the same place so that if a physician is moved to a different room, she will know exactly where to find the common items. A specific drawer in each room could be stocked to accomplish the same outcome.

=======================================*FAST FACTS in a NUTSHELL*

- Supply management starts with stocking rooms efficiently and effectively.
- A commonality between rooms will reduce the time looking for supplies during patient care activities.

A consistent system and identifying one person as being responsible for ordering can eliminate the frustration of being without a supply at any given time. Usually in smaller clinics, one of the nursing staff takes on this responsibility. In larger clinics, supplies are usually maintained by a separate department. Selecting the right person is crucial to controlling costs with medical supplies. If a physician wants a new gadget or supply, a procedure should be followed prior to the supply being ordered. Sometimes it is important to order that once-in-a-lifetime product. You want the supply orderer to think the process through prior to ordering.

A consistent system may include a chalkboard or posted list in a key place to identify items needed. When a nursing staff takes the last item, they write down the item needed. Use of a designated trash can for all empty supply boxes could also work, especially if you have varying individual items. The supply clerk could write down the item using the box instead of guessing what item is needed.

Supply ordering can be done in numerous ways: in person, online, or by phone. Comparing prices on a regular basis is crucial. Have a set of items you frequently use priced by a different vendor at least once every six months, or check different sources when you need a specialty item. There are numerous medical supply discount pricing companies that can be joined to get reduced pricing on medical supplies. Most hospitals are associated with a discounted buying organization and can include physician practices as part of their group.

===*FAST FACTS in a NUTSHELL*

- Ordering supplies can be streamlined by having one person responsible for this task.
- Supply ordering can be done online, in person, and over the phone.

Durable medical equipment (DME) supplies, such as orthotics or crutches, are stocked in physicians' office for patient convenience. Reimbursement should be fully explored prior to offering this service. The above stocking guidelines will provide consistency and efficiency with DME as well.

Supplies can become outdated, so rotating stock is required. Packaging that is turning yellow or other items in less-than-perfect condition should be discarded. Organizing supplies for ease of use can take some thought, but will be much appreciated when the item is needed.

===*FAST FACTS in a NUTSHELL*

Rotation of supplies will prevent the need to discard old items.

Coordination of Care

Many nursing activities are performed after the patient leaves the practice. These include managing physician orders, coordinating the patient care with other health care providers, pre-authorization, coding, arranging for testing, paperwork, and managing pharmaceutical representatives.

It is important to establish how physician orders will be handled in the practice before problems arise. Too often, it is assumed that nursing staff and physicians have talked about parameters, and then a physician is shocked when it is brought to his attention that his nurse gave a certain prescription. The procedure should include answers to the following questions:

- Who can place orders? Nurses only, unlicensed personnel, doctors only
- How are orders transmitted? Fax, verbal, sent with patient
- Are there standing orders? Who can use them and when?
- How are prescriptions renewed? By pharmacy, patient, fax, phone, electronically?
- Can nursing staff renew prescriptions for certain medications?
- Can the nursing staff use the physician's stamp for certain orders?
- Can the nursing staff initiate certain treatments?
- Can the nursing staff give out samples if the patient asks for them?
- How current does the patient have to be for a medication to be refilled?

Other order issues include verbal orders and physician stamps. Verbal orders can be tricky for a medical office. Limiting the use of verbal orders by requiring the nursing staff to fax any orders with the physician's signature on it limits misunderstanding and reduces exposure.

A physician stamp is commonly used in a physician's office. A procedure and physician's approval for its use should first be obtained. The procedure may indicate that a stamp can be used for orders for lab and radiology, referrals to outside agencies or outside health care providers (home health, DME, etc.), or for claim filing. The physician should specifically indicate how the stamp can be used. It is always a good idea for the person who uses the stamp to also provide their initials after it to indicate the stamp's authenticity.

Because of the nature of the job, nursing staff sometimes need to initiate treatment without obtaining consent from a physician. For example, a patient calls in with a cough that has been persistent for several weeks. Because he has worked with this physician for many years, the nurse knows that the physician will want to see a chest x-ray before seeing the patient. A chest x-ray is ordered. This scenario saves the physician time. However, just to prevent potential problems, there should be a list of protocols that the nursing staff can follow that the physician has signed off on. This also allows other staff to work with a physician in the absence of his nurse. Remember that when that nurse orders a chest x-ray, she is actually practicing medicine without that written document.

Coordinating patient care across the health care continuum is often the role of the nurse. In many ways, if the relevant information is at the nurse's fingertips, she will be more efficient. A cheat sheet that includes a list of all community resources, names, and phone numbers will speed up the nursing staff in making those calls. This can be separated by physician preference.

Providing information to referral sources and hospitals will help better coordinate patient care. A system should be developed that automatically initiates a procedure when the patient is sent to the hospital or a referral physician. The procedure should include what information should be sent and when. Another system should be in place for information that returns to the practice after the patient sees the referring physician, is hospitalized, or was seen in the emergency room. Electronically, this can be tracked with open orders and closing the loop when the information has been obtained. A paper log can be created to track the same things as well.

In some offices, nursing follows the specialist into the hospital setting with procedures or surgeries. Scheduling at multiple locations is a challenge at times. Blocking time for one physician or a group of physicians makes this somewhat easier if they can sustain the volume. If there is not an option for blocking time and the physician would like to go to multiple locations, care should be taken to schedule at one specific location for a given period. One surgery office was struggling with this, and a physician was scheduled at three different locations in one morning. It was agreed that the physician would be scheduled at one location after that location was first scheduled. In other words, the first patient who wants to go to location 1 on a Thursday, for example, means that any other patients who want to see that physician on that same Thursday must also go to location 1. The physician also agreed to visit two locations in the same day, so the day often was divided between the two locations. This was much better than the three locations in one morning that he was accustomed to previously. His production increased substantially.

Another coordination activity involves coding. To ensure proper and easier coding, the nursing staff should meet on a regular basis with a coder or someone who understands coding. A simple cheat sheet created by the coder of the most frequently used codes can be helpful. Also, having a resource that you can call if you have any questions can be an efficient way to complete some tasks.

With all of the different insurance company requirements, the nurse needs to know which insurance companies will allow which labs. If there is any way to make this easier by choosing a lab that takes all insurances (in a perfect world), the nurse's job becomes much easier. In lieu of that, a cheat sheet that lists the insurance company and the lab required is a necessity. If diagnostic testing can be approved electronically, either by fax or through the computer, time is saved. Talk to the testing sites and see if this is an option.

Another problem with diagnostic testing is that the testing center needs a diagnosis accompanying the ordered tests. A cheat sheet can be created to assist the nurse in the major diagnoses he may use when ordering tests. Pre-authorization may be needed for certain radiology tests. Working with the testing center when approving a given procedure is most often successful. They want your business and will help make it easier for you to refer patients to them.

If a diagnostic test is ordered, results should be tracked to ensure they are received. Any liability carrier will tell you there is great risk in not following up on tests ordered. This can be done in numerous ways, but it takes commitment from the nursing staff to ensure it is complete. Various ways include:

- The nurse keeps the chart until the test result is received.
- A tracking log kept by an individual or group with the date noted as to when the results were received. This works well if all test results come into one location, such as a fax, fax server, or mail.
- A copy of the order is kept until the results are obtained.

Nursing staff may also have to track tests that are ordered yearly (e.g., mammograms and colonoscopies). Most practice management systems have this capability to track and/or generate a letter as a reminder. A small card file works well for an individual physician to set up tracking. Registries can also be used to create a list of patients who require preventive care.

Many procedures or surgeries require pre-authorization, depending upon where the procedure is performed. This is an important item for the billing office, but doesn't carry the same importance for nursing staff. For that reason, if possible, this should be placed in the hands of the billing office. A hand-off sheet can be created to assist in ensuring that the billing office has all the information needed.

Organization is needed to make sure patients are given access to reduced prescription costs. Nursing staff will tuck away things given to them, but often have to search to find these items when that once-a-year case comes along. Make it easier on them by organizing a book so that they can go promptly to the right pharmaceutical company and give the patient the appropriate forms. The book becomes a reference in helping patients. Once again, due to the complexity of this task, one designated person may need to take on this role.

Patients will hand the nursing staff numerous types of paperwork to be filled out for their employer, insurance company, etc. A clear policy on how this process works is important. In one practice, the nursing staff instructed the patient to return to the front desk, pay a nominal fee, and then the nursing staff filled out the paperwork. Paperwork never reached the nursing staff until the fee was paid.

Pharmaceutical representatives can create a bottleneck in a medical office. Most often, the way in for these drug reps is through the nursing staff. If you have a timid or friendly nursing staff, your physician may be in trouble. The reality is that nursing staff control access to their physician. A clear policy is needed for any practice, whether it is "no drug reps" or defined times when drug reps can be seen. It is also helpful to give assertive response training so that staff know the appropriate words to use. As salespeople, reps can sometimes be difficult to get rid of. Citing a policy with regard to reps can make it easier for staff to deal with them.

Efficiency for the nursing staff is tied to other office staff: the front desk, billing, phone attendants, and physicians. Having a collaborative approach to working together makes everyone more efficient and everyone will provide better patient care. Working to problem-solve patient or workflow issues is a win-win for all.

======*FAST FACTS in a NUTSHELL*

- Coordination of care involves many aspects and tasks.
- Coordination of care includes all other nursing duties.

CAPITALIZING ON TECHNOLOGY

Technology is becoming more prevalent in a medical office, and it can either hinder or enable the nurse. Sometimes, when technology is brought into a situation, we tend to just place it on top of already created workflows. In order to use technology effectively, however, the workflow sometimes has to be redesigned.

Understanding current processes can be accomplished simply by writing it down. Take a bulletin board, a white board, or even a blank wall using sticky notes and start by listing all steps in the process. Each individual step can then be explored as to whether it is necessary or whether it adds value to the whole process. Duplicate steps can be found, and a more efficient process can be created. This process works the best if people who work in different areas of the practice sit down together and talk about what each one's responsibility is in the process. For instance, the receptionist who checks the patient into the practice may be taking time to ask about allergies, and the nursing staff is unaware of this step. The nursing staff could then be asking the same question. Although it takes only a few moments to do this, those few moments add up if multiplied by 20, 30, or 100 patients per day.

Technology is not always the right thing to add. Looking at the benefits it will bring to the practice or to your role and to the patient is the first step. Looking at the workload and weighing that against the benefits can also help determine if it is the right step.

FAST FACTS in a NUTSHELL

- Nurses add value to the medical office for many reasons.
- Understanding the differences between RN functions and nonlicensed nursing duties can maximize both roles.
- Many efficiencies can be realized in nursing functions.

9

The Future of Medical Office Nursing

INTRODUCTION

After reading this book, you now can make a decision as to whether medical office nursing is right for you. The future of medical office nursing is vast and wide open for creating a truly rewarding career. This chapter will look at several new and upcoming thoughts and directions for this career.

In this chapter, you will learn:

1. Different possibilities for medical office nursing roles.
2. Trends in nursing roles and a rediscovery of the role of the RN.

THE FUTURE MEDICAL OFFICE

Many new models of care are being piloted to improve efficiency and change outcomes in medical offices. Primary care has been striving to improve the work and satisfaction of physicians for several years, and some new and exciting models are emerging. Technology has taken on a life of its own in the medical office, and it will affect future care in many different ways. Managing the entire patient population and providing care in new care management models is showing promising rewards right now. Health care reform is happening now, and will have an impact on nursing. This section takes a look at the future.

Patient-Centered Medical Home

In early 2000, the leading physician organizations for family medicine, internal medicine, and pediatrics created a list of principles that would need to be implemented if primary care was to survive in the future. The number of primary care physicians is declining, as are the residents who are interested in primary care. Primary care physicians accumulate the same debt after medical school as specialists and then go to work for much less money. Therefore, many potential primary care physicians choose instead specialty care to seek higher wages and better working hours.

The principles that were created and agreed upon led to more interest in taking care of the entire patient through a continuous relationship with a primary care physician, providing more access, managing patients across a continuum, and using technology effectively. The name for all of this was the "patient-centered medical home."

The "medical home" concept was created by pediatrics forty years ago to help take care of chronically ill pediatric patients in a more comprehensive manner. This same concept is now being applied in various forms to many primary care specialties.

Primary care practices throughout the nation are testing this new model of care through pilot programs led by insurance companies and large, integrated delivery systems. It is starting to catch on and create an excitement in the primary care community. Reimbursement is being tested with these pilot programs to pay for quality and care management/care coordination in addition to paying per visit as the current system allows.

The patient-centered medical home creates a medical office environment that is focused on the patient and on developing a continuous relationship with a primary care provider. It focuses on patient access to that provider through appointments, e-mail, or phone for acute, preventive, and chronic needs. The primary care provider provides care management and care coordination for his panel of patients to better manage their conditions across the continuum. Evidence-based medicine is stressed and incorporated in the day-to-day operations so that care is delivered consistently and effectively. The use of technology helps to improve the efficiency of the practice. The health care team provides a collaborative relationship with the patient to engage them in management of their health care needs. Managing the practice more efficiently and effectively leads to better quality care and outcomes in a variety of areas: financial, clinical, and satisfaction of providers, staff, and patients.

This can be expanded to other health care providers, such as hospitals, specialists, and community agencies, to collaborate and coordinate the patient's care. The patient remains at the center of care, and all efforts are tailored to facilitate better health. This concept stresses the importance of relationship building. The patient builds a relationship with the primary care physician, who collaborates with referring providers and other agencies (including hospitals) to take care of the patient in a comprehensive manner.

Although the name is somewhat limiting, the concept of providing more efficient, cost-effective care is here to stay. Focusing on evidence-based medicine instead of experience-based medicine can lower health care costs and provide better outcomes. The RN's role in the medical home is evolving, with particular attention on care management and care coordination, which is expanded on in the following sections.

=========================*FAST FACTS in a NUTSHELL*

The patient-centered medical home is emerging as a new model of care that can affect satisfaction, access, and patient involvement with their primary care physician.

Increased Use of Technology

Most industries have made the technological leap, and health care is now being asked, and sometimes shoved, to do the same. There is no question that electronic technology can change and improve care delivery. Physician offices have been slow to adopt the technology because of several factors. In particular, many systems have not grasped the true essence of care and the eloquence of the physician-patient relationship.

Many technology leaders fail to understand that having the physician do more does not help in delivering care. For instance, in a traditional office, the phone call is routed to the nurse or medical assistant. The medical chart is pulled, and the message is written down. If the physician needs to be consulted, the nurse leaves the medical chart on the physician's desk for review and to answer the question presented. In the world of technology, the receptionist takes a message, which is oftentimes routed to the physician without any triaging assistance by the nurse. This can be true for lab results, prescription refills, and any documentation that arrives at the practice. Also, physicians who are used to dictating may now find that they have to spend time clicking through boxes and typing into the record. Thus, they have taken on administrative tasks. The physician's workload has doubled at a time when her most important task is to see and treat patients.

Technology companies need to realize that just because the task has been made easier for the practice, oftentimes it has multiplied the workload of the physician. The use of the team is important in streamlining only those items that require the physician's knowledge and skill and directing them to him. Thinking about those processes and how the EMR will change them is important when deciding whether to implement this technology. If an EMR is in place, looking at all the responsibilities of the physician, and determining the need for his expertise versus someone else on the team doing this is the key in making technology work for the practice.

================ FAST FACTS in a NUTSHELL

- Technology use is increasing in medical practices.
- A review of all processes prior to implementation will improve efficiency.

New technology is emerging daily for both the clinical and administrative portions of the practice. New EMRs, registries, patient portals, chronic disease portals, and endless other tracking and clinical documentation advances are being tested. The design of the exam room and how technology can be incorporated to improve efficiency are also being tested. New surgical and specialty offerings occur on a regular basis. The interaction between tools in the office and the EMR has already been initiated at many levels. Much progress can be expected as physicians realize the potential of automation and point-of-care technology.

New technology is also emerging for other parts of the practice that will affect nursing. The ability to complete referrals or pre-authorizations online instead of having a paper form to fill out is the start of automating insurance connections. Ordering tests through a portal, instead of having a lab requisition them, and having tests return to the office without staff touching paper are some of the advances that will spur even more innovations.

Technology is probably the biggest and greatest improvement that we will see over the next decade as medical practices try to catch up with the technology revolution. The development of better user interfaces, transfer technology, and telecommunications technology are just a few of the areas we might see vast improvements in. Accessibility of data will be a key driver to improve outcomes and reduce cost.

═══════════════════════════════*FAST FACTS in a NUTSHELL*

The growth of new technological advances will be seen in the future medical office

Care Management

Our population is aging, and there is an increasing number, severity, and duration of chronic illness. Lifestyle has a large impact on chronic disease in the form of obesity and smoking habits. Ambulatory care has become the setting for chronic disease management. There is a growing shift from acute and chronic episodic care to care management with a focus on population management. New programs are being created to work with chronically ill patients to try to curb the costs by better managing their care.

In addition, there is a shift towards controlling health care costs and improving quality. Although U.S. health care spending outstrips that of other countries, certain outcomes lag far behind. This has led to employers and businesses stepping into the health care debate. More effectively managing overall patient care is quickly becoming the more prevalent strategy suggested by insurers, employers, and the government. Medicare and Medicaid are moving towards a more quality-driven reimbursement method as they require providers to define, measure, and assess quality in the care they provide.

This is a huge opportunity for nurses and nurse practitioners to work as care managers or case managers in many aspects of ambulatory care. Health education and health promotion are still not reimbursable expenses, but they play a vital role in maintaining the health of a population.

A wide range of knowledge is required to manage more complex chronically ill patients. A team including nurses, pharmacists, social workers, physicians, nurse practitioners, and other providers will need to work together to find and carry out solutions. Collaboration among specialists, hospitals, and disciplines will have to be the norm instead of the exception to coordinate patient and population care needs.

=====*FAST FACTS in a NUTSHELL*

There is a growing shift from acute and chronic episodic care to overall care management of the patient population.

Other Aspects

In health care, there is a heightened awareness of the increased power of the consumer to participate in health care decisions. As patients become more knowledgeable about their disease or condition, they can take a more active role. Increasing interest in disease prevention and health promotion will spur further development of consumer-driven alternative prevention and therapies to complement mainstream medicine. Nurses can help drive and educate patients as they become more engaged in their own health care.

TRENDS IN THE NURSING ROLE

There are an increasing number of roles for ambulatory care nurses in many aspects of the health care picture, from the insurer to the medical office:

- Nurses will provide patient education and work with chronic disease patients to manage their illnesses more effectively. Perhaps incentive programs will be created to reward those nurses with the best outcomes as nursing's role is better realized.
- Nurses will be asked to take a greater role in technology as health care becomes more technologically advanced. Nurses can play a key role in development, customization, and support for health information technology due to their knowledge of the clinical aspects of care. Telenursing, including remote monitoring, is just emerging as an area that could be further developed and specialized. Virtual care is just now being realized. Online clinics may be in the future, and nurses may play a larger role working over the phone.

- Roles in quality improvement and outcome measurement are sure to follow the increased focus in this area.
- Case management roles will be more prevalent as outcome measurement and chronic illness care develops. The case manager, who usually works for the insurer, will develop the plan of care for the complex, high-utilization patients and work with team members to enhance quality of care and reduce cost across a variety of settings. They assess the patient, develop a plan of care, and evaluate the outcomes. Often, case managers become involved with catastrophic illnesses such as cancer or end-of-life care.

=*FAST FACTS in a NUTSHELL*

There are many new and exciting roles for nurses in ambulatory care.

One role that hasn't been mentioned but has been underlying all ambulatory care development is nursing leadership. Moving into uncharted territories and developing new roles will require nurses to step up and lead. From the nurse who cares for the patient on the phone to the nurse manager or administrator who oversees clinical operations, there is a need for more sophisticated nursing managers and leaders in the medical office setting. Medical office nursing requires clinical experience and strong communication skills. Knowledge of financial and reimbursement systems, as well as business expertise, is needed to effectively and efficiently manage care.

Nurse leader competencies include:

- Technological skills, which facilitate mobility and portability
- Expert decision-making skills
- Ability to create quality and patient safety cultures
- Appropriate intervention in health care debates
- Collaborative and team-building skills
- Ability to envision professional nursing in the ambulatory care setting
- Use of research findings to provide better care to patients
- Ability to react to a rapidly changing health care environment

An educational support system that teaches and develops leaders to move through this time of change will assist the ambulatory care nurse to flourish. Nurses are needed as educators in all aspects of ambulatory care as well as educators of nursing staff.

=====*FAST FACTS in a NUTSHELL*

Nursing leadership is a key component of the future of nursing in ambulatory care.

REDISCOVERING THE ROLE OF THE RN

There is a myth that nurses in medical offices could not "cut it" in the real world and therefore they chose ambulatory care. This image is changing rapidly with the complex management of chronically ill patients; patients are not staying in the hospital for as long. Nurses require more specialized education and training in critical care skills to manage patients. Critical thinking and clinical judgment are required at all times with telephone triage and telehealth monitoring. Often, nurses are providing time-constrained phone assessments of a critically ill patient and making instant decisions.

In many instances, only one RN is present in an office setting, and this role requires an ever-increasing need to demonstrate independent thinking skills. Delegation to nonlicensed assistants requires knowledge of supervision, understanding roles, and new skill sets. The comprehensiveness of the RN role allows for flexibility and ingenuity. Nurses are needed in the medical office.

================= *FAST FACTS in a NUTSHELL*

- The future medical office is being developed now by piloting new methods of care.
- Technology will play a key role for nursing in the future.
- Many new roles are emerging for nursing in the medical office.

DEFINITIONS

- Accounts receivable: Money that is owed to the practice for services provided to patients from numerous sources, including patients, insurance companies, and government payers.

- CPT (Current Procedural Technology): A numeric code used to identify specific services provided.
- Care management: Identifying and managing specific patient groups by engaging the patient in prevention and management of chronic illnesses.
- EOB (explanation of benefits): A statement from the insurance company explaining payment of services.
- EMR (electronic medical record): A software program that allows all clinical aspects of the patient visit to be documented.
- Encounter: A patient's face-to face visit with a provider.
- ICD-9 (International Statistical Classification of Diseases): A numeric code that is used to identify diseases and symptoms.
- Medical service: Any care provided by health care providers.
- Nonlicensed staff: A person who provides care in the office but is not regulated or licensed by a state regulatory board.
- Patient panel: A group of patients assigned to a physician.
- Practice management system: A software program that provides administrative functions for a medical office, including scheduling, billing, and reporting.
- Portal: An online tool that gives the patient the ability to communicate with the practice in the form of e-mail or structured messaging.
- Population management: The ability to provide proactive care to a group of patients.

ADDITIONAL READING

1. U.S. Department of Health and Human Services, Centers for Medicare and Medicaid Services, Medicare Learning Network. Evaluation and Management Services Guide. Retrieved November 11, 2009, from http://www.cms.hhs.gov/MLNProducts/downloads/eval_mgmt_serv_guide.pdf
2. National Quality Forum. *National Voluntary Consensus Standards for Ambulatory Care*. Retrieved November 21, 2009, from http://www.qualityforum.org
3. Centers for Medicare and Medicaid Services. *2010 Physician Quality Reporting Initiative List of Measures*. Retrieved November 23, 2009, from http://www.cms.hhs.gov/PQRI/Downloads/2010_PQRI_MeasuresList_111309.pdf
4. Richmeier, S. (2010). *Leading Your Clinical Team: A Comprehensive Guide to Optimizing Productivity and Quality*. Englewood, CO: Medical Group Management Association.
   (Various aspects of Chapter 8 have been adapted from this book.)

Index